W9-CZT-909

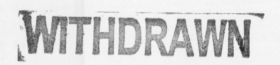

WITHDRAWN

St. Louis Community College

Library

5801 Wilson Avenue
St. Louis, Missouri 63110

Physical Activities for the Handicapped

PHYSICAL ACTIVITIES
FOR
THE HANDICAPPED

MARYHELEN VANNIER

Southern Methodist University

PRENTICE-HALL, INC., *Englewood Cliffs, New Jersey*

Library of Congress Cataloging in Publication Data

VANNIER, MARYHELEN, (date).
    Physical activities for the handicapped.

    Includes bibliographies.
    1. Physical education for handicapped persons.
2. Handicapped—Recreation. I. Title.
GV445:V25   790.19'6   76–9750
ISBN 0–13–665638–2

10 9 8 7 6 5 4 3 2 1

PRENTICE-HALL INTERNATIONAL, INC., *London*
PRENTICE-HALL OF AUSTRALIA, PTY. LIMITED, *Sydney*
PRENTICE-HALL OF CANADA, LTD., *Toronto*
PRENTICE-HALL OF INDIA PRIVATE LIMITED, *New Delhi*
PRENTICE-HALL OF JAPAN, INC., *Tokyo*
PRENTICE-HALL OF SOUTHEAST ASIA PTE. LTD., *Singapore*

This book is dedicated to the blind children
with whom I work as a volunteer recreation leader,
in gratitude to each one
for helping me see more fully the beauty, joy,
and wonder of life.

Contents

▌▌ The Problem 35

III   **The Program   127**

Preface

This book is first of all a presentation of a wide range of physical activities for the handicapped, their place and the contributions they can make in the rehabilitation and education of the handicapped. Secondly, it is a book of methods for teaching and leading these atypical people successfully through many kinds of well-conducted physical activities in a school or recreational setting.

It has been written mainly for two groups: (1) college students who are preparing for careers as professional physical educators or as special education teachers, and (2) those who are working as therapeutic recreation specialists conducting physical activities for the handicapped in a variety of settings within the community.

The author, who has had wide experience teaching professional preparation programs in physical education and recreation on the university level as well as working directly with exceptional children and adults afflicted by many different kinds of handicaps, believes that good leadership and teaching methods can be mastered by those who really want to learn them. She also strongly believes that sports, games, and other types of physical activities should play a much larger role in the life of the handicapped, for through such activities people of all ages can find challenge, satisfaction, beauty, and joy in life.

The concern for bettering the lives of the millions of handicapped persons upon this earth has never been greater than it is now. Those entering this challenging field as professional leaders or as volunteers must be dedicated in their desire to help every handicapped person attain a more joyous and productive life.

The author is indebted to many persons who helped with the preparation of this book. She is especially grateful to all who submitted photographs and other materials used in this publication and especially to Dr. Julian Stein, AAHPER; Benjamin Lipton, National Wheelchair Athletic Association; Lyonel Avance, Special Physical Education Project, Los Angeles City Schools; Ted Moulton, Principal of the Northlake Elementary School of Richardson, Texas; Maudie Warfel, of the National Foundation of Happy Horsemanship for the Handicapped; Lane Goodwin, of Wisconsin State University; Dr. Charles Buell of the California School for the Blind in Berkeley, California; and to Norman Acton of Rehabilitation International in New York City.

MARYHELEN VANNIER

1

BACKGROUND

The handicapped child has the right to grow up in a world which does not set him apart, which looks at him not with scorn or pity or ridicule but which welcomes him, exactly as it welcomes every child, which offers him identical privileges and identical responsibilities.

From the report of the White House Conference on Child Health and Protection, Committee on Physically and Mentally Handicapped

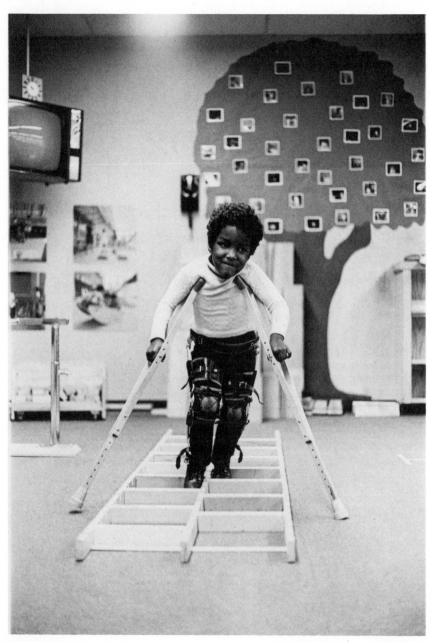

Determination is a greater factor in gaining mastery of physical skills or other kinds of learning tasks. Courtesy of the Richardson, Texas Public Schools.

1

Physical Educational and Recreational Programs for the Handicapped

In America, attitudes toward the handicapped are changing rapidly. Up until the seventeenth and eighteenth centuries, the blind, deaf, crippled, and anyone else who did not look or act "normal" were regarded as evil creations of the devil. They were often destroyed, hidden away in caves, or left on mountain tops for wild beasts to devour. Even today some people still fear the handicapped, yet often view them with morbid curiosity. During the early American colonial period, epileptics were chained to stakes, the insane were thrown into snake-filled pits, and the blind, deaf, crippled, or retarded were either destroyed at birth or hidden away in dark rooms by their guilt-filled parents.

How fortunate we human beings are that throughout the history of mankind there have always been a few courageous people who have devoted their lives to help others less fortunate. Since the coming of Christianity there has slowly developed throughout the centuries a concern for the individual human being regardless of his physical or economic condition and racial heritage. In our country from its earliest beginning there were a few such people who sought help for all the unfortunates, including the handicapped. However, it was not until the period between 1817 and 1850 that real impetus and strong leadership was given to the concern for the health, vocational, and educational welfare of exceptional people. Such leaders as Horace Mann and Samuel Gridley not only spoke out in behalf of the retarded, they actually began the first educational programs for them. Dorothea Dix was among the first to spark public concern, with resulting preventive and corrective programs, for socially

3

maladjusted children. In 1817 Reverend Thomas Gallaudet established the first American school for deaf children. The Massachusetts School for the Blind and the still famous Perkins Institute for the Blind came into being in 1929. They were soon followed by the establishment of more schools for the deaf scattered throughout the nation. Oddly enough, it was not until decades later that schools for deformed and crippled children became a reality.

At the turn of this century, public awareness of the many problems of the handicapped gradually became a reality. World Wars I and II, in which thousands of young men were rejected from military service because of physical disabilities or were left crippled as a result of combat, became turning points in the development of special programs devised around the special needs of the handicapped. "Normal" individuals who returned as disabled persons in need of help caused fellow citizens to look upon them as human beings worth assisting in the community, at home, and in the labor market. Soon after curative workshops and rehabilitation centers were established for these handicapped adults, the parents of exceptional children began to unite to find aid for their own offspring. Thus, in 1940, the United Cerebral Association came into being, owing largely to the determined efforts of a small group of dedicated parents of brain-damaged children. The success of this group heartened the parents of mentally retarded children, who organized and conducted fund-raising campaigns on local, state, and national levels. From their efforts, the National Association for Retarded Children soon came into being. The National Conference on Mental Retardation conducted in 1956 by the U.S. Department of Health, Education and Welfare was a result of one of their goals. Since then, vast sums of money have been provided for teacher education, research, demonstration centers, and clinics for the mentally retarded. As one authority has pointed out, parental timidity has given way to action programs, and interest has expanded into almost every facet of the many problems of exceptionality, including needed medical research, legislation, and program innovations.[1]

Today increasing attention is being focused upon the handicapped person of all ages and types. Throughout the country there are now many fine programs in the following areas:

1. Physical therapy—correction of remediable defects brought about through therapeutic exercise programs based upon the recommendations of a physician.
2. Recreational therapy—the handicapped helped to develop social and physical skills through such activities as sports and games, arts and crafts, music and drama, and other recreational outlets.
3. Corrective therapy—physical exercise programs designed by physical

---

[1] William Cruickshank and Orville Johnson, *Education of Exceptional Children and Youth,* 2nd ed. (Englewood Cliffs, N.J.: Prentice-Hall, 1967), p. 11.

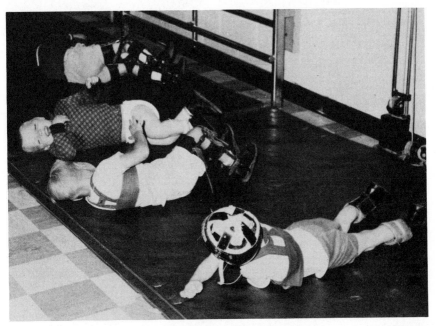

All children should have chances to take part in rolling activities as a means of learning body control and directionality. Courtesy of the AAHPER.

education specialists presented on an individual or small-group basis in schools, camps, or rehabilitation centers.

4. Special education—the school curriculum modified to meet the needs of the exceptional; specially trained teachers working with special kinds of equipment either at school or as visiting teachers to provide students with educational services often into postschool life.

5. Adapted physical education—physical activities such as rhythms, sports, and games modified according to the special physical problems of an individual or a group of students.

6. Developmental physical education—those below normal in stamina, motor coordination, or endurance taking part in physical activities under the direction of a specialist in order to correct specific physical weaknesses.

7. Corrective physical education—changes or improvements brought about in body structure and function through exercises designed by a physician or corrective specialist.

8. Rehabilitation and reconditioning physical exercise programs—begun during World War II; veterans confined to hospitals helped through physical exercise programs; field now known as physical medicine include patients of all ages; e.g., stroke and/or accident victims, etc., who are in need of such programs.

9. Habilitation programs—handicapped individuals taught how to take care of the physical needs found in daily life in their home environment

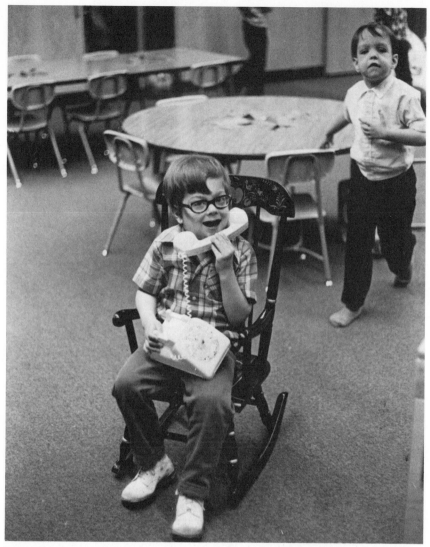

By using miniature models, the handicapped can often learn the many skills needed to live in our modern society. Courtesy of the Richardson, Texas Public Schools.

and at work, such as performing household duties, learning how to drive a car, etc.

10. Occupational therapy—a certified therapist working as a member of a medical team carrying out an individual plan for each patient in order to obtain desired objectives, such as helping the patient learn how to relax, find recreational outlets for social development, or learn prevocational skills.

Since the turn of the century, our federal government has become increasingly concerned about developing programs in the areas of health, education, and welfare for all citizens, including the handicapped. Public Law 90-170, passed in 1967 and titled "The Training of Physical Education and Recreation Personnel for the Mentally Retarded and Other Handicapped Children," provided for advanced professional preparation of physical education and recreation specialists in various universities as well as for the establishment of research projects and demonstration centers in both physical and recreational activities for the atypical.

Within the near future, more and better trained personnel will become available to fill the needs of the handicapped as a result of these and other professional preparation programs. There will also be stepped-up programs in both research and demonstration centers, resulting not only from the passage of Public Law 90-170 regarding the handicapped but also from the important three-day Study Conference on Research and Demonstration Needs in Physical Education and Recreation for Handicapped Children. This conference, jointly sponsored by the American Association for Health, Physical Education and Recreation, the National Recreation and Park Association, and the Bureau of Education for the Handicapped of the U.S. Department of Health, Education and Welfare, was held at the University of Maryland in February 1969. The outcomes of the conference were: (1) the identification of major problems needing to be studied, (2) the setting up of research priorities, and (3) the development of dissemination methods so that research findings could be centrally housed, shared, and fully utilized.

It is through such meetings and programs as these that existing physical education and recreational programs for the handicapped will be upgraded, many more new ones will come into being, many problems will be faced and solved, and long-range working plans and goals for the future will be established.

WHO ARE THE HANDICAPPED?

In one sense of the word, there are times and situations in which everyone may be handicapped. For example, an American in Russia would be handicapped socially if he or she could not communicate verbally. Often the words "exceptional," "special," or "atypical" are used interchangeably with the term *handicapped*.

The victims of physical and mental disabilities and diseases lack the capacity to compete with the normal and generally have emotional and social adjustment problems. These persons fall into two classifications: (1) the physically handicapped and (2) the socially handicapped. Within these two groups, each individual differs widely, for no two of these persons are alike any more than any two normal human beings are.

Types of physical handicaps are:

Postural	Speech
Crippling	Respiratory
Visual	Cardiac
Hearing	Nutritional
Convalescent (from illness or injury)	Epileptic, tubercular, and endocrine
Asthmatic and diabetic	disorders

Types of social handicaps are:

Feeblemindedness or mental retardation
Social maladjustment and emotional disturbance

Some authorities believe that the mentally gifted should also be listed as being socially handicapped. Certainly this would be true if no special provisions were made for them in all phases of the school curriculum, including physical education, as well as in the home, neighborhood, and community.

It is estimated that in America, which now has a population exceeding 200 million, there are approximately 50 million Americans who have emotional, intellectual, or physical handicaps. Of this number, over 13.5 million are children and youth. Conservative estimates indicate that 10 to 12 percent of all our public school children and youth at the present time are emotionally disturbed and need psychiatric help. As Dr. Joseph Douglass of the National Institute of Mental Health has pointed out,

> Our nation has phenomenally high rates of infant mortality, malnutrition, birth defects, juvenile crime, emotional illness, chronicity and physical impairment, among other problems.
>
> If our entire male population of draft age were examined, approximately one-third would be disqualified for military service. Hearing, language and speech disorders occur in 15 percent of our population under 21. Also, approximately 22 percent of the clients served under vocational rehabilitation programs are under the age of 20.[2]

The most common handicaps found among public school children and youth are congenital defects, cardiac conditions, cerebral palsy, those resulting from polio, accidental injuries, epilepsy, cancer, osteomyelitis, tuberculosis, and diabetes.[3]

It has long been known that children and youth who are nonwhite in low-income groups are often the most permanently damaged. Those living with migratory parents, those in ghettos, or those in inner cities are least likely to have defects corrected. Many are labeled as mentally retarded when they actually have faulty vision or cultural deafness (a technique of tuning out the noise of many persons living in close quarters in slum conditions). The seriousness of overcrowding, the population explosion, inadequate medical care, and lack of income are now being recognized as serious national economic and cultural problems. It has been estimated that 20 to 40 percent of all school children in our present society suffer from one or more chronic conditions. As one authority has pointed out, about 30 percent of these handicapping conditions could be prevented or corrected through good medical care during the first five

---

[2] "Is Man Free to Make Choices for Health?" *School Health Review*, 7 (September 1969), p. 5.

[3] Richard Kraus, *Therapeutic Recreation* (Philadelphia: W. B. Saunders, 1973), p. 7.

years of life, and if care could be continued to age 18, as much as 60 percent of all found defects could be corrected.[4]

It is estimated that between 5 and 10 percent of all school children should be in some program in special education. Table 1–1 shows the handicaps by which these children are classified.

Table 1–1   Classification of Handicaps

Handicap	Percentage
Low physical fitness	20 to 25
Poor body mechanics	50 to 60
Nutritional disturbances	1 to 2
Visual handicaps	1 to 2
Auditory handicaps	1 to 2
Cerebral palsy	less than 1
Cardiac conditions	1
Arrested tuberculosis	less than 1
Diabetes	less than 1
Anemia	less than 1
Asthma and hayfever	2 to 4
Hernia	less than 1
Epilepsy	less than 1
Mental retardation	1
Other	1

Source: Hollis Fait, *Special Physical Education: Adapted, Corrective, and Developmental,* 3rd ed. (Philadelphia: W. B. Saunders, 1966), p. 10.

The needs of the exceptional can be met if the following points are recognized:

1. Their needs are practically the same as those of normal persons.
2. They can usually profit more from being with normal groups than from being segregated; they need to be encouraged to mix with those who are normal.
3. Normal children can often help them to recognize their limitations and to work around them. Although children are often cruel, they accept any handicapped child who proves he has licked his problem and can do many other things better than they can.
4. Few can be helped to any great extent who have been too sheltered by parents who have allowed them to remain helpless over a long period of time.
5. All need to solve their own problems, to take and assume responsibilities, and to have good friends to help them become adjusted to their own limitations, environment, and society.

4 Douglass, "Is Man Free to Make Choices for Health?" p. 6.

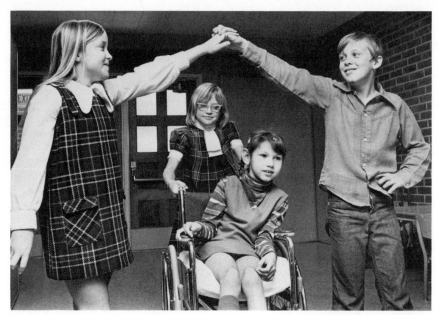

Handicapped children and normal children have much to learn from each other. Courtesy of the Tucson Public Schools.

6. Work and play programs must be geared to their limitations, environment, and ability, yet be challenging enough so that the children can
and will progress.

RECREATIONAL PROGRAMS
FOR THE HANDICAPPED

Increasingly, public recreation departments, community organizations, voluntary youth-serving agencies, and church groups are providing
recreational and educational programs for the handicapped of all ages.
All such programs, to be most successful, must be planned and conducted
in terms of each individual participant's needs, interests, and capabilities.

Because many handicapped persons leave special schools before the
age of 18, they frequently lack both knowledge of existing programs and
the means to get to them. Consequently, there should be surveys made
within communities to determine the actual number and location of
exceptional people and a well-organized effort to provide them with
information and adequate transportation.

A good program should include such activities as the following: [5]

---

[5] See the appendices for recommended equipment for both large- and small-group
instruction and therapy.

Dramatic and Language Activities
  debates
  pantomime
  panel discussions
  puppetry
  play acting
  publication of a newspaper
  skits
  story telling and writing
  variety shows
  poetry reading

Arts and Crafts
  basketry
  beadcraft
  carving wood, soap, brick, bone
  ceramics
  costume design
  jewelry making
  millinery and dressmaking
  model airplanes, cars, trains, villages
  painting
  photography
  woodworking

Dance
  ballet
  folk
  movement exploration
  modern
  social
  square

Special Holiday Celebrations
  Hallowe'en
  Thanksgiving
  Christmas
  New Year's
  4th of July
  Valentine's Day

Table Games
  bingo
  card games
  checkers
  chess
  dominoes
  puzzles

Sports and Games
  baseball
  basketball
  bowling
  golf
  handball
  horseback riding
  roller and ice skating
  sailing
  skiing
  soccer
  swimming
  table tennis
  track and field for elementary school
    children
  tumbling
  volleyball

Music
  singing
  glee clubs
  instrumental groups
  record listening

Nature and Camping
  astronomy
  bird watching
  campcraft activities
  caring for and training pets
  fishing
  gardening
  hunting
  mountain climbing
  nature study

Service Projects
  care of facilities
  care and repair of equipment
  typing and mimeographing
  life guarding
  shopping for supplies
  meal planning and cooking
  setting tables, serving, and clean-up
    of food
  making clothes or other articles for
    the needy

The Therapeutic Recreation Leader

In addition to the desirable character qualities and leadership skills of all recreation leaders, those working with the handicapped through the media of recreation must:

1. Not feel sorry for those handicapped and let them learn to do things for themselves
2. Have an abundance of patience and a rich sense of humor, imagination, and creativity
3. Be able to reach each individual within each group, helping him to gain social and communicative skills as well as to be a good citizen
4. Be willing, if necessary, to deal with such things as the feeding, lifting, toilet, and transportation needs of the handicapped
5. Be in good physical, mental, and emotional health

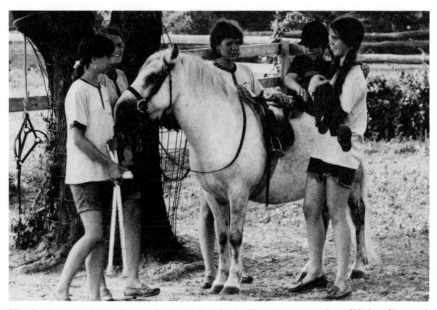

The leader must be understanding and be physically strong enough to lift handicapped children as well. Courtesy of the National Foundation for Happy Horsemanship for the Handicapped, Inc.

There are many types of therapeutic recreational specialists who work with the handicapped to help them to regain or improve their health, overcome or work around their disabilities, and assume responsibility for their own future as much as possible. These leaders are found in a variety of settings working with people of all ages who have many kinds of disabilities. Some are counselors in camps for handicapped children, others are recreational therapists in hospitals, institutions, or nursing homes, while still others work with homebound "shut-ins," or at government rehabilitation centers. Regardless of title (whether it be occupational, physical, corrective, dance, music, art, or play therapist), this leader is a valuable member of a team headed by medical personnel. His or her responsibilities vary depending upon the setting and the job.

However, the duties of the activity leader usually include the following:

- Conducting a wide variety of program activities ranging from arts and crafts through many kinds of sports and games
- Organizing large-group entertainment-type activities such as a bingo game or a community sing
- Keeping and requisitioning needed supplies and equipment
- Attending in-service training sessions, staff meetings, and conferences
- Writing reports and case studies
- Contacting outside agencies for such things as trips and entertainment
- Conducting in-service training sessions for volunteer and assistants

The leaders must be able to understand diagnostic information and be skilled in selecting exercises, games, and other recreational activities that will help each patient improve health as well as physical and social skills. The cooperation of many people is needed to conduct a program of merit.

SPECIALIZED PHYSICAL EDUCATION FOR THE HANDICAPPED

The exceptional individual is first of all a human being, and secondly, a person with some unique kind of a handicap. Although most exceptional people are acutely and painfully aware of their physical limitations, almost all of them are totally ignorant of their physical development potentialities.

Until recently, many schools excused atypical students from physical education classes. Those with only slight handicaps were often allowed to do such things as keeping score during activities. Such practices are apt to do more harm than good. *All* children need to learn how to play and to be taught basic body control and movement skills. The unskilled child, if he is further handicapped by being physically disabled, is in for a lonely, isolated, unhappy future. It is through specially devised physical education programs that thousands of handicapped individuals are being educated to face and realize their limitations and to learn how to work around them.

Today there are three basic kinds of specialized physical education programs: adapted, corrective, and developmental. Adapted physical education is a modification of physical activities according to the physical limitations of an atypical individual or group. Corrective physical education is a program of specific exercises and activities designed to improve body mechanics when standing, sitting, or moving through space. Developmental physical education is concerned with the improvement of the physical fitness and motor coordination of those who are below established standards as measured by various diagnostic tests.

All exceptional persons should be encouraged and required to take part in the physical education program, just as are all normal individuals.

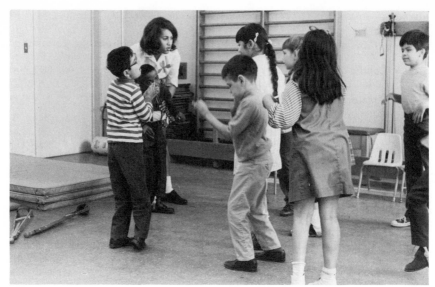

The adapted physical education class can be made up of students with a wide variety of handicaps. Courtesy of the Los Angeles Public Schools.

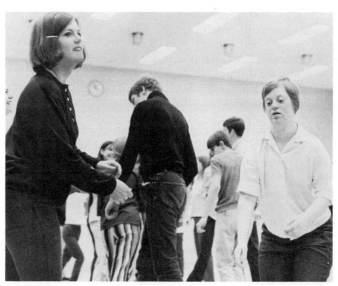

The adapted physical education teacher knows that handicapped children can learn much more than most people think they can. Courtesy of the AAHPER and Lane A. Goodwin.

Following are points to be remembered by the teacher in charge of the adapted, corrective, and/or developmental physical education program.

1. The program must be built upon the individual needs of each child.
2. The program must be conducted under the supervision and direction of a recognized medical authority.
3. The teacher should have specialized professional preparation to be able to do this work successfully.
4. The parents' cooperation must be sought and secured.
5. The students should follow the same procedures and rules in as many things as possible in normal groups, including class participation, costumes, and grading.
6. Classes for severely handicapped children should be kept small. The kind of defect will determine grouping possibilities. Malnourished children, for example, can have classes with those suffering from cardiac and respiratory defects.
7. Pupils should be assigned to special classes according to the amount of physical work permitted.

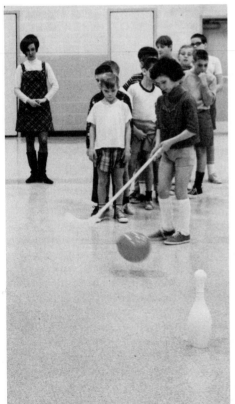

Learning to play according to rules and to take turns is an important thing to know. Courtesy of the AAHPER and William H. Daniels.

8. Complete records should be kept for each student, including results of the physical examination, health history, observation and data from family, reports sent to other staff members, a record of behavior, and personality rating.

9. The program should be set up in the gymnasium or a room large enough for adequate equipment. The following minimum items are recommended:

> stall bars
> mats or mattresses with washable covers
> scales
> individual benches without backs
> flying rings
> bulletin boards
> individual exercise cards
> filing cabinet for records
> screens
> cots
> full-length mirrors
> punching bags
> iron boots
> horizontal ladders
> knee, ankle, and leg exercisers
> muscle-testing instruments
> recreational games

The Specialized Physical Education Teacher

In addition to a knowledge of and skill in teaching needed for successfully conducting a wide variety of physical activities, a teacher working with the atypical should have a vast understanding of the human body, first aid, and the causes, nature, and effects of handicapped disabilities. This person must have a basic understanding of human behavior as well as a "feel" for teaching and people. Most crucial is (1) the patience to work with exceptional individuals (because their progress in learning skills is often painfully slow) and (2) total acceptance of such pupils (because many of them may be repulsive looking and even grotesque). The more one knows about individual pupils and their particular handicaps, the more successfully one can reach and teach them. Parent conferences will prove helpful; if they are well planned there will be a feeling of rapport, support, and willingness to work together. Such conferences can help the teacher establish controls necessary for protecting students from physical or emotional injury.

Horace Mann, the famous American educator, once declared that "the teacher who is attempting to teach without inspiring the pupil with a desire to learn and improve himself is hammering in vain upon cold iron." John Ruskin believed that "education does not mean teaching people what they do not know. It means teaching them to *behave* as they do not behave." Actually the primary purpose of any educational experience is to help each learner attain completeness as a human being. Though these basic beliefs about teaching and learning are educationally sound, they are only of merit if they shape the attitudes and sharpen the sensitivity of the teacher as students are patiently guided, molded, and motivated. It is the leader who is the key to bringing about behavior change that is called "education."

PUBLIC RELATIONS AND COMMUNITY SERVICES

Educators are increasing their attempts to interpret educational and recreational programs for the handicapped to the tax-paying public. They realize that although these programs are costly, the public will give support for the handicapped, as well as the normal, if a need for such programs exists. It is, then, of vital importance that the general public be fully informed concerning existing or needed programs for handicapped adults and children.

Establishing Objectives

Although the average person is usually aware that handicapped people need medical attention and educational programs tailored to their difficulties, many do not know of the importance of providing physical activities programs for them as well. Many adults, especially those in rural areas, still regard recreation as an expensive frill or even sinful. Therefore, the public relations effort is extremely important if such programs are to continue and be supported by the public.

Basic to planning a good public relations program is deciding (a) *what kind* of a publicity program is needed, (b) to whom it should be directed, (c) what it aims to accomplish, and (d) how to evaluate its effectiveness.

One authority in recreation for the atypical has suggested that the objectives of the public relations program might well be:

1. To interpret the need for and benefits of recreation for the handicapped
2. To inform handicapped individuals concerning the program being offered and to enlist them as participants so that a greater number may benefit from these available sources
3. To enlist volunteers to help in the program
4. To secure financial support necessary for the establishment or continuance of the program as well as to secure needed equipment and supplies
5. To give the community an accounting of the work being accomplished in recreation for the handicapped
6. To share information concerning recreation for the handicapped with

related agencies, organizations, and groups interested in the handi-capped [6]

All publicity should be geared to reach these above objectives. Tim-ing is an important factor in releasing all publicity, whether it be to campaign for additional funds or to entice more volunteer aid. Accuracy of information is of vital importance.

Often the best means of publicizing any recreational or educational program is through "satisfied customers." However, this type of scattered publicity should be coupled with all centralized public relations en-deavors. Some organizations hire public relation experts to plan and carry out a continuous yearly publicity program.

Publicity Media

The variety of media for publicity includes demonstrations, exhibits, television and radio broadcasts, newspaper articles, brochures and other kinds of printed materials, and public speakers.

DEMONSTRATIONS FOR THE PUBLIC

A demonstration for the general public (given preferably at night so that more can attend) should be an outgrowth of some regular program. It should show such things as (1) activities learned during the year; (2) a hobby group's accomplishments; (3) pupil demonstrations followed by participation in activities by the parents; or (4) activities built around a general theme such as physical fitness.

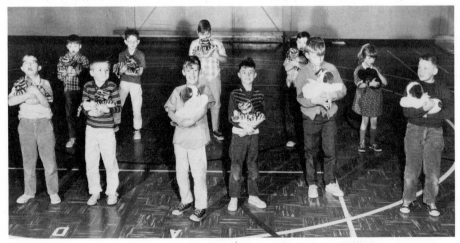

Demonstrations for the public constitute one type of public relations. Courtesy of the AAHPER.

[6] Janet Pomeroy, *Recreation for the Physically Handicapped* (New York: Mac-millan, 1964), p. 111.

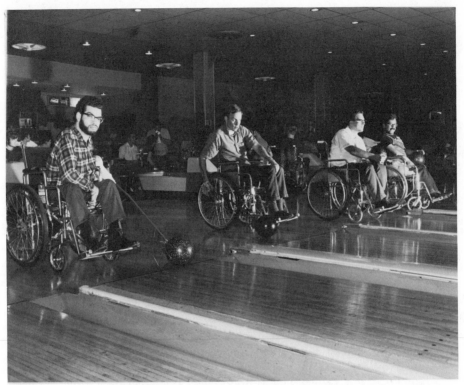

Competitive events held at public facilities help acquaint the general public of your program. Courtesy of the National Wheelchair Athletic Association.

It is very important that all members of the handicapped group take part in a public demonstration, for this will make it a more meaningful experience for parents, friends, and community members. Committees that can be formed to help organize demonstrations might be the following:

The program committee: Theme selection, who will participate and what each will do, featured events, procession and recession, the grand finale, the complete program in its entirety

The publicity committee: Use of newspaper publicity, spot announcements for radio and television stations, fliers, responsibility for printed or mimeographed programs

The facilities and equipment committee: Bringing and returning all needed equipment, checking the public address system

The hospitality committee: Welcoming and seating all spectators

The clean-up committee: Performing all necessary janitorial duties

A planning committee composed of the leader and an elected representative from each group should be responsible for the entire demonstration. All those in the program should evaluate their results with the leader when it is over. Their specific recommendations for future programs should be filed and referred to for the planning of future programs.

EXHIBITS

Colorful exhibits of an arts and crafts program can do much to help the general public learn that the handicapped can be creative and productive. Such exhibits should be placed where they can be seen best. They may be in the form of posters, snapshots, paintings, or table displays of articles made by the participants.

TELEVISION AND RADIO PROGRAMS

Because radio and TV are required by law to provide public service programs, they offer many opportunities to promote activity programs for the handicapped. This publicity may be in the form of spot announcements, live interviews, or complete programs from the recreation center or special school. Any publicity should be both concise and informative.

NEWSPAPERS

Human interest stories written by professional journalists can do much to awaken the general public to the needs of the atypical person. Because newspapers often stress the unusual, they may overemphasize the emotional side of news items in order to play upon public sympathy rather than presenting a factual well-balanced version of a story. This likelihood can be lessened if the leader prepares interesting, accurate information which will become the heart of the printed article. The use of photographs will enhance reader interest. Permission should be obtained for the reproduction of all materials.

Newspapers prepared by the handicapped provide both recreational outlets for group members as well as good publicity. The most economical method of producing such a paper is mimeographing it. The paper would have a variety of news items and might well include sports, social activities, announcements of coming events, a gossip column, engagements and marriages, and a poetry section. Classified advertising space can be sold to underwrite the cost of producing the paper, if necessary.

BROCHURES AND OTHER PRINTED MATERIALS

Brochures should be concise and informative. The use of color and photographs will increase reader interest. They should be printed in clear type, bordered by many white spaces. Copies of those distributed by the American Heart Association or the Epilepsy Foundation of America can be secured to use as models by any organization wishing to develop brochures of their own. A fact sheet can also be used to convey much information briefly to those seeking it. This announcement should include the time the facilities will be open for meetings or classes, program offer-

SUNSHINE COMMITTEE TO PHONE ABSENTEES

The HH Sunshine Committee is accepting responsibility for calling members who, for a month or more, have not been present at the Center.

Any member who, for reasons of security, wishes to be "checked on" may leave his name at the office to be turned over to Chairman MAE NORWOOD.

Five members have been added to the committee. They are EULA HUFFHINES, FEROL WRIGHT, LEE McCOMB, IVAN HARRELL, and HATTIE MAE STEVENS.

MYSTERY TRIP PLANNED!

Do you like surprises? Would you like to be one of those happy-go-luckies who don't know where they're goin' but are on their way? If so, the HH Mystery Trip is just for you!

The group will be made up of the first 46 persons to sign up (and pay up) at the office. Only the date, April 7, the time of departure and return, 9 and 1:30, and the cost, $3.25 will be revealed! Oh, yes -- one other item--LUNCH is included in the $3.25 charge!

The DESTINATION ??????????????????
Why not take a chance? Columbus did!

IF YOU WANT TO KEEP YOUR CREDIT UP PAY YOUR MONEY DOWN!

Registration fees for this year were due January 1, with a period of grace extending to February 1. Those not paying by that time, unless by prior arrangement, have been automatically dropped. A charge of $1.00 is charged for reinstatement.

This rule was made necessary by the fact that each year a considerable number of members have been several months delinquent in paying their registration fees. No business could be operated efficiently under such conditions, and neither can HH!

In cases of hardship or financial problems the staff is always willing to make concessions.

"It is one of the most beautiful compensations of this life, that no man can sincerely try to help another without helping himself."
                                    Shakespeare

If we noticed little pleasures as
  we notice little pains,
If we forgot our losses, and remembered all our gains,
If we looked for people's virtues,
  and their faults refused to see,
What a comfortable, happy, cheerful
  place this world would be!
            From THE NEW ENGLAND ADAGE
            Submitted by Louise Campbell

SILENT TONGUE

Sometimes our kindest deed can be ... To say not any word ... As when there is a rumor or ... Some gossip we have heard ... Our silence then is golden and ... It will be better yet ... If we ignore the statements and ... Endeavor to forget ... There is a time and place to judge ... A critical report ... An authorized committee or ... A fair judicial court ... It is so wrong to pass along ... The smallest tale or two ... Even if we have cause to think ... The information true ... The gossips spit their poison out ... When they have drained the cup ... Whereas they would be better off ... If they would just shut up.
                                    Anonymous

DRAMA GROUP IN THE MAKING

Does HH have any would-be actors and actresses among its members? The Reverend Stephen Love has offered to direct a Drama Group and/or a Play Reading class. If this sounds like something right up your alley, please fill in the coupon below and return to the HH office.

I would be interested in a Drama Group_____
I would be interested in a Play Reading Class_____
NAME_____
PHONE #_____

Fig. 1-1 A Sample Newspaper Written by a Group of Senior Citizens at Hospitality House in Dallas, Texas

To: Dallas Senior Citizens
Subject: Hospitality House

WHAT IS HOSPITALITY HOUSE?

1. An ACTIVITY DAY CENTER offering recreational, cultural, educational, and services to the community ACTIVITIES – with the philosophy that one is never too old to learn.
2. OPEN MONDAY through FRIDAY, 9:00 a.m. to 4 p.m.
3. A DEPARTMENT of THE SENIOR CITIZENS FOUNDATION OF DALLAS (RI 1-5416)

WHERE IS IT LOCATED?

1. 5111 Capitol Ave., Dallas, Texas (Educational Building MEMORIAL UNITED METHODIST CHURCH)
2. TELEPHONE NUMBER: 827-3911
3. MAILING ADDRESS: 5111 Capitol Ave., Dallas, Texas 75206

WHO CAN BELONG TO HOSPITALITY HOUSE?

1. RESIDENTS of Dallas County WHO ARE 55 YEARS OF AGE OR OVER who are PHYSICALLY and MENTALLY able to participate in group activities and help in management.
2. PERSONS who enjoy good fellowship, good times, and the opportunity to share the creative experience of learning new skills as well as practicing old ones.

HOW TO BECOME A MEMBER OF HOSPITALITY HOUSE:

1. COME to Hospitality House THREE TIMES.
2. EACH TIME, sign the YELLOW PROSPECTIVE MEMBER SHEET.
3. On your SECOND VISIT, ask the RECEPTIONIST for an APPLICATION FORM.
4. On your THIRD VISIT, bring the COMPLETED APPLICATION form to the HH OFFICE and make an appointment to see the HOSPITALITY HOUSE DIRECTOR.

WHAT IS THE MEMBERSHIP REGISTRATION FEE?

1. Minimum fee is usually $5.00; maximum fee is unlimited. Membership is renewable each January 1st. No one is denied membership because of inability to pay $5.00. Membership is paid yearly.

WHO CAN VISIT HOSPITALITY HOUSE?

1. Visitors of any age can visit ONCE and must REGISTER on the BLUE SHEET.
2. EACH MEMBER may invite ONE GUEST per month and WILL REGISTER him/her on the BLUE SHEET, giving GUEST'S NAME and HIS OWN NAME.

HOW IS HOSPITALITY HOUSE SUPPORTED?

1. Yearly grant from the E.D. Farmer Foundation to The Senior Citizens Foundation.
2. Donations from individuals, churches, and civic groups.
3. Membership registration fees.
4. Memorial gifts.
5. Donations from Hospitality House Members.
6. Sales sponsored by the HH Members (Bake, Clothing, White Elephant, etc.)

Fig. 1-2 A Sample Fact Sheet

ings, the location of the center, school or other facility, as well as other needed information (see Figure 1–2).

SPEAKERS

Talks given to civic groups, the PTA, clubs, and other organizations also serve as excellent ways of interpreting programs for fellow citizens. Because the effectiveness of this type of communication depends solely upon the skill of the speaker, only people who can convey messages well should be chosen to speak to outside groups. The use of color slides or movies can contribute greatly to the listeners' interest and help them develop a wider understanding of the program.

In this chapter we have reviewed the basic physical activities programs for the handicapped and stressed the need to keep the public informed and to involve them in promoting and providing these programs within the community.

SUGGESTED READINGS

Bureau of Education for the Handicapped, *Physical Education and Recreation for Handicapped Children,* A Study Conference on Research and Demonstration Needs. Washington, D.C.: American Association, for Health, Physical Education and Recreation, and National Recreation and Park Association, 1969.

CRUICKSHANK, WILLIAM, and G. ORVILLE JOHNSON, *Education of Exceptional Children and Youth,* 2nd ed. Englewood Cliffs, N.J.: Prentice-Hall, 1967.

DAUGHTERY, GREYSON, *Methods in Physical Education for Secondary Schools.* Philadelphia: W. B. Saunders, 1967.

FAIT, HOLLIS, *Special Physical Education: Adapted, Corrective, and Developmental,* 3rd ed. Philadelphia: W. B. Saunders, 1972.

FRYE, VIRGINIA, and MARTHA PETERS, *Therapeutic Recreation: Theory, Philosophy, and Practices.* Harrisburg, Pa.: Stockpole Books, 1972.

KRAUS, RICHARD, *Therapeutic Recreation Service.* Philadelphia: W. B. Saunders, 1973. Also *Recreation and Leisure in American Society.* New York: Appleton-Century-Crofts, 1971.

NESBITT, JOHN, PAUL BROWN, and JAMES MURPHY, *Recreation and Leisure Services for the Disadvantaged.* Philadelphia: Lea & Febiger, 1970.

POMEROY, JANET, *Recreation and the Physically Handicapped.* New York: Macmillan, 1964.

SHERRILL, CLAUDINE, *Adapted Physical Education.* Dubuque, Iowa: Brown, 1976.

STEIN, THOMAS, and H. DOUGLAS SESSOMS, *Recreation and Special Populations*. Boston: Holbrook Press, 1973.

VANNIER, MARYHELEN, and HOLLIS FAIT, *Teaching Physical Education in Secondary Schools*, 4th ed. Philadelphia: W. B. Saunders, 1975.

WEISKOPF, DONALD, *A Guide to Recreation and Leisure*. Boston: Allyn and Bacon, Inc., 1975.

2

Programs
of the Handicapped

Parents of a handicapped child often face severe and longlasting psychological and social problems. As their child grows older, many of these problems increase in intensity. Parents of an epileptic offspring often fear "crossing" him, believing that such action would bring on a seizure; thus the child soon gains an upper hand and becomes almost uncontrollable both at home and school. Many handicapped young children can play successfully with a few peer friends but, as they grow older, are

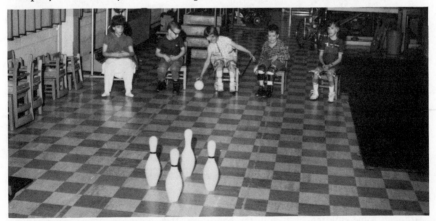

Many handicapped children are lacking in social as well as physical skills. Courtesy of the AAHPER and the University of Iowa.

quickly dropped as a playmate because of their inability to keep up. Because the atypical child is so often unable to compete in athletic contests, he loses a good chance to gain peer status through active games and sports. Moreover, his various therapeutic treatments may require so much time that he often has difficulty keeping up in school. As an adult he is faced with the challenge of finding employment and a marriage-partner. For many such individuals life is a tremendous struggle that is damaging to physical, emotional, and educational development.

Those who suffer from multiple disabilities (such as cerebral palsy combined with mental retardation and blindness) are the most severely handicapped of all, and the number of severe and/or multiple handicaps

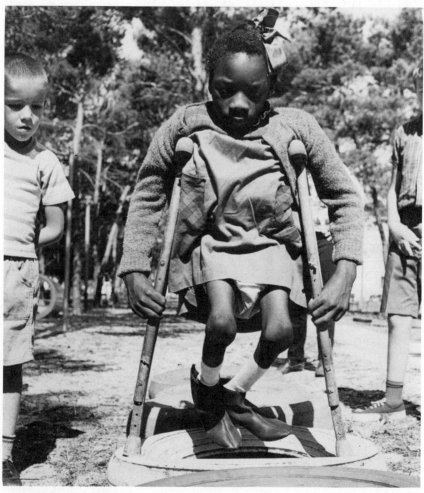

Although some children have multiple handicaps, they have the same basic emotional needs as normal children. Courtesy of the AAHPER.

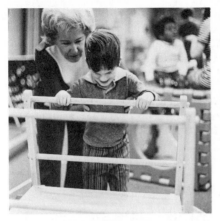

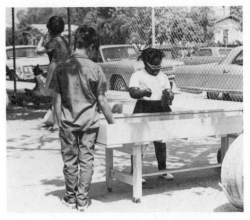

Children who gain teacher acceptance have a higher opinion of themselves and are more outgoing. Courtesy of the Richardson, Texas Public Schools.

Every person needs to have a good friend with whom to talk and share many kinds of other experiences. Courtesy of the Los Angeles Public Schools.

is increasing at a rapid rate throughout the world, owing largely to the population explosion.

The greater the severity of brain damage, the greater the decrease in performance and movement accuracy, and the greater the personal adjustment problems. Although most handicapped children benefit from being within learning and social situations with "normal" children, however, there are certain exceptions and qualifications. It would not help either the normal or the handicapped, for example, in the case of children so severely retarded as to be minimally trainable; contact with the normal population is assumed and necessary, obviously, only in their care and maintenance. But even the most badly *physically* handicapped individuals need positive contact with the real world. (This, of course, involves helping normal children to learn how to deal humanely and constructively with others who are perhaps grotesquely deformed.) In certain handicaps, such as blindness, special teaching within the disabled group only is a necessity for dealing with specific learning problems; but closeness to the normal population must be maintained in other learning situations, because the blind must learn how to live within the normal world. Those children disabled in cardiac functions usually do well with normal children in most kinds of personal-social situations involving self-appraisal. But far too many handicapped people live tragically lonely lives and are social outcasts.

PHYSICAL PROBLEMS

In a 1960 study conducted by 166 physicians in New York City child health stations, and involving 22,873 children, the three most frequently found disease categories were respiratory, skin and allergy, and hernia and muscular. The results of this study are shown in Table 2–1. It was also found that 39 percent of all children examined had one or more adverse health condition. Many of these children were badly handicapped at birth.

Table 2–1 Survey of Children Examined by Physicians in New York City Health Stations for Well-Child Care (New York City Department of Health, October 1956–May 1957)

	Conditions Diagnosed and Rate per 1,000 Children Examined by Ethnic Group							
	White		*Nonwhite*		*Puerto Rican*		*Unknown*	
Condition	*No.*	*Rate*	*No.*	*Rate*	*No.*	*Rate*	*No.*	*Rate*
Respiratory	812	135	1,334	137	1,054	176	127	112
Skin, allergy	424	71	886	91	337	56	93	82
Hernia, muscular	72	12	829	85	96	16	71	63
Genitourinary	65	11	364	37	313	52	49	43
Infections	156	26	193	20	162	27	27	24
Orthopedic	131	22	235	24	107	18	31	27
Nutrition	89	15	197	20	146	24	24	21
Congenital malformations	146	24	138	14	127	21	15	13
Dental	170	28	102	10	66	11	19	17
Diseases of the blood	61	10	57	6	119	20	15	13
Emotional, behavior	54	9	69	7	50	8	14	12
CNS-eye	49	8	77	8	48	8	6	5
Gastrointestinal	36	6	93	10	44	7	7	6
Trauma, accidents	22	4	45	5	31	5	7	6
Neuromuscular, mental	26	4	44	5	26	4	8	7
Cardiovascular (nonorganic)	24	4	42	4	19	3	6	5
Cardiovascular (organic)	18	3	33	3	28	5	8	7
CNS-speech	20	3	14	1	7	1	2	2
Metabolic	7	1	13	1	13	2	2	2
Convulsive seizures	9	1	7	1	8	1	2	2
Cancer, leukemia, tumors	7	1	6	1	10	2	—	—
CNS-ear	2	*	1	*	—	—	—	—
Miscellaneous	23	4	33	3	27	5	9	8
Total	2,423	403	4,812	494	2,838	474	542	477
No. of children examined	6,008		9,740		5,989		1,136	

From James Wolf and Robert Anderson, *The Multiply Handicapped Child*, 1960. Courtesy of Charles C Thomas, Publisher, Springfield, Illinois.

* Less than 0.5 per 1,000.

In this study it is significant to note that the results showed that:

1. In health matters, there was a significant ethnic difference between white and nonwhite groups.
2. There was a much higher incidence of hernia and muscular conditions among the nonwhite.
3. A significantly higher number of males had adverse health conditions than females.
4. Orthopedic conditions were the sixth most frequently diagnosed disorder. These abnormalities ranged from club foot to rheumatoid arthritis.
5. Nutrition was the seventh most common disorder found. Obesity was seen much more frequently than malnutrition.
6. The most frequently found gastrointestinal disorders were diarrhea, gastroentertis, colitis, and acute appendicitis.

Although these findings should not be interpreted as representing frequency of adverse health conditions of all children and infants in our society, they do clearly show that persons in lower socioeconomic groups have far more serious health problems than others, and that children in the under–18-month age category have higher percentage of serious health problems than the 18-month and over group.

A child who deviates from normal both in appearance and function often develops major social and emotional problems which basically are due to a physical problem. The correction and elimination of such problems is basic to the reduction and elimination of the problems of social acceptance and emotional health.

THE FAMILY

The greatest influence in the life of a handicapped person usually is his family, for the child tends to look upon his disability the same way his family does. Many parents may be oversolicitous and shield their handicapped child too much; those who do not will be more likely to have a well-adjusted offspring who is aware of his strengths as well as his weaknesses and limitations.

Until recently, many parents refused to acknowledge the existence of an atypical child as a member of the family. Those who were severely mentally retarded, cerebral palsied, or epileptic were often hidden away by their families. Guilt feelings frequently haunt parents of handicapped children. Most parents today, however, work honestly and openly for their disabled children's benefit. But it is still a rare family that can plan adequately for a happy, realistic future for its handicapped child without the help and counsel of professionals.

Factors that often cause nonacceptance by the community, such as a child's grotesque or crippled appearance, can cause serious family problems. A child with epilepsy often has a higher degree of social rejection

than a child with a vision impairment. Those with mild mental retardation are usually well-accepted by their families and society in contrast to
those who are severely crippled or mongoloid. The larger the number
and the greater the degree of multiple handicaps, the more likely are the
chances for parental and community rejection and disharmony. The
handicapped child must not only adjust to society and his own limitations,
he also must strive for acceptance by his family and peers.

It is of great importance for the handicapped child to feel accepted
within his family from the very beginning of life. Nonverbal communication, such as the way he is held or talked to by either parent, soon conveys
to the child that he is loved and wanted or despised and rejected. As he
learns to cope with speech, movement, and behavior problems, he also
gains self-discipline and a clearer understanding of himself. One problem
closely related to a negative family relationship has to do with the parents'
methods of dealing with the problem of the handicap. Often parents tend
to be overprotective and do too much for the child, such as buttoning
his clothing, combing his hair, or not letting him run and play with peers.

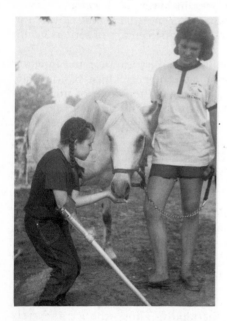

Caring for a pet can be a therapeutic experience for any handicapped person.
Courtesy of the National Foundation
of Happy Horsemanship for the Handicapped, Inc.

If the parent teaches the child from an early age to be independent, to
do things for himself, to accept and work around his limitations, that
child is off to a good start and is most likely to develop into a self-supporting, capable human being in adulthood. This assumes a good family
relationship, usually.

In short, although sibling rivalry is often a problem among all
children, among the handicapped it often becomes more serious, especially
if others in the family feel that they have been demoted to a lesser place
in the eyes of their parents.

THE SCHOOL

Extreme care must be taken to make school experiences positive ones for the handicapped child. The teacher must not only accept the child and his limitations, she must also help her other students to gain respect for this person too. As Fait points out,

> In developing a favorable climate in the classroom for the acceptance of those who are physically or mentally handicapped, the teacher may discuss with the students the reasons for liking and disliking certain people. The importance that is sometimes attached to attractive physical appearance may be pointed out and contrasted with more meaningful personal attributes. In connection with this point, it might be emphasized that performing the best one is capable of is just as admirable and worthy of respect as being the most outstanding performer. Attention should be directed toward the concept that one does not have to play well the popular spectator sports such as football and basketball; success, according to one's ability, in an adapted game of corner ping pong or loop badminton is of no less significance than success in the more popular games.[1]

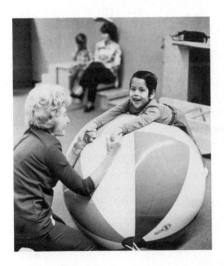

The physical therapist is a vital part of a rehabilitation team. Courtesy of the Richardson, Texas Public Schools.

If possible, the child should be placed in a corrective or developmental physical education program conducted by a specialist in this field if he lacks coordination, physical strength, and overall fitness. His program should be made up largely of specific exercises and games selected to correct and/or eliminate physical difficulties. If the student is placed in an adaptive program, activities should be offered that will lead to better leisure-time use as well as provide him with opportunities to gain physical skills such as accuracy in aiming and timing, or improved hand-eye or foot-eye coordination.

---

1 Hollis Fait, *Special Physical Education: Adapted, Corrective, and Developmental* (Philadelphia: W. B. Saunders, 1966), p. 16.

The Guidance Program for Parents

There is a pressing need for close cooperation and understanding between the home and school if an exceptional child is to realize his optimum growth and development. There should be a guidance program for parents which involves physicians, ministers, psychologists, social workers, and teachers. Such a program is best located in a consultation center. The physician should be the key person in the guidance team. If the child is enrolled in school, this major person should be the principal or the special education expert. Frequently it is this teacher working closely with the school administrator who can help the parents to focus more clearly upon their child's limitations and needs for special instruction.

Parent Groups

Parent groups made up of those who have adjusted well to having a handicapped child have a significant role to play in helping other parents accept help, and adjust to having such an offspring. Such groups gain mutual strength and support because members share the same kinds of problems. Under strong leadership these groups can also become powerful forces for the betterment of the exceptional, both at school, within the community itself, and even nationally.

In the school setting, parents usually work as teacher helpers. Many seek recreational outlets for their children from other community agencies such as the city recreation department. Often parents assist in such programs by serving as teacher-leaders, being on the board of directors of agencies interested in helping the handicapped, or by providing transportation. Those who become teacher-leaders should not work with their own child, for he or she can gain independence and peer status better when placed in a group that is not directly involved with family.

Parent Conferences

There may be times when a conference designed to learn more about and give further help to a handicapped person should be a parent-teacher-pupil meeting. Often, however, the conference should be a meeting between only the parents and teacher to check on the child's progress, discuss mutual problems, and develop a closer relationship so that they can work as a team for the child's benefit. The conference should be followed by a visit in the home of the child, if at all possible. The teacher should make the initial step by establishing a meeting time either through a note or phone call. Other suggestions for the teacher are:

1. Plan conferences in advance with *all* parents.
2. Tell the parents the aim of the conference.
3. Expect and welcome *both* mother and father at parent conferences.

4. Be friendly, interested, relaxed, and to the point.

5. Accept and respect the parents.

6. Listen to what parents have to say.

7. Try to find out all you can about the child without prying.

8. Be completely honest.

9. Begin and end in a positive manner.

10. Have representative material of the child's work, a fair sampling containing examples of both good and bad work to show parents.

11. Have physical test information in lay language to give to the parents.

12. Have the child's cumulative record on hand for reference.

Some cautions for the teacher in such a conference are:

1. Don't try to confer with parent when either parent or teacher is emotionally upset.

2. Don't try to crowd a conference into too short a time.

3. Don't try to cover too much material.

4. Don't compare the child with other children or with brothers or sisters in his family.

5. Don't try to "out-talk" the parent.

6. Don't quote capacity or mental ability (IQ) test scores to parents.

7. Don't make conferences too formal.

8. Don't alarm parents with "norms," "means," or other statistics of a professional nature which they may not understand.

9. Don't repeat any personal material.

10. Don't sit behind the desk if at all possible, but rather sit in a chair facing the parents.

Above all, the establishment of good rapport is of vital importance, so that all parties concerned can unite in the goal of providing the best possible kind of developmental environment for the child.

SUGGESTED READINGS

American Foundation for the Blind, *Services for Blind Persons in the United States*. New York: The Foundation, 1960.

BARBE, W. B., *The Exceptional Child*. Washington, D.C.: Center for Applied Research in Education, 1963.

CRUICKSHANK, W. M., "The Multiply Handicapped Cerebral Palsied Child," *Exceptional Children*, 20 (October 1953), 16–22.

DELACATO, C. H., *The Diagnosis and Treatment of Speech and Reading Problems*. Springfield, Ill.: Charles Thomas, 1963.

GINOTT, HAIM, *Between Parent and Child*. New York: Collier-Macmillan, 1965.

———, *Teacher and Child*. New York: Collier-Macmillan, 1972.

HUNT, J. M., *Intelligence and Experience*. New York: Ronald Press, 1961.

JENKINS, GLADYS, *Helping Children Reach Their Potential*. Chicago: Scott, Foresman, 1961.

KILLILEA, MARIE, *Karen* (1953); *The Love From Karen* (1965). Englewood Cliffs, N.J.: Prentice-Hall.

MAGARY, J. F., and J. R. EICHORN, *The Exceptional Child, a Book of Readings*. New York: Holt, Rinehart and Winston, 1969.

National Easter Seal Society for Crippled Children and Adults, "Prejudice and Rehabilitation of the Socially Handicapped," *Rehabilitation Literature*, 32, No. 1 (January 1971).

WHEATLEY, GEORGE, *Health Observation of School Children*. New York: Mc-Graw-Hill, 1965.

WILLIAMS, MARIAN, and HERBERT LISSNER, *Biomechanics of Human Motion*. Philadelphia: W. B. Saunders, 1962.

WOLF, J. M., *The Blind Child With Concomitant Disabilities*. New York: American Foundation for the Blind, 1967.

WOLF, JAMES, and ROBERT ANDERSON, *The Multiply Handicapped Child*. Springfield, Ill.: Charles Thomas, 1969.

WRIGHT, B. A., *Physical Disability, A Psychological Approach*. New York: Harper & Row, 1960.

THE PROBLEM

Man wanders over the restless sea, the flowing water, the sights of the sky, and forgets that of all wonders, Man himself is the most wonderful of all.

The Dallas Health and Science Museum

3

Mental Retardation

In Chapters 3, 4, and 5, we will deal with three separate types of handicaps, giving each a separate chapter because of their importance and frequency. In the chapters following, several disabilities will be discussed within individual chapters.

As a group, the mentally retarded are more normal in the area of motor activities than in any other. However, some individuals within this group are markedly behind others in the areas of body control, movement accuracy, and the ability to maintain balance while moving or changing directions quickly. Some are unable to understand directions. Cratty has found trainable *mentally* retarded children and youth to be much lower in performance than *educable* retardates in the areas of body perception, gross body agility, locomotor agility, and throwing skills.[1] Other studies have shown the retarded to be far behind normal children in hand dexterity skills and fine motor coordination. Improving in motor control can, through physical education, help the retardate to more easily cope with his normal peers, improve his effectiveness as a worker, aid in his enjoyment of life, and stimulate his growth in communicative and social skills.

Mental retardation is a growing national problem. In 1960 there were an estimated 5.5 million mentally retarded people; according to

---

[1] B. J. Cratty, "The Perceptual Motor Attributes of Mentally Retarded Children and Youth," Monograph, Mental Retardation Services Board of Los Angeles County, August 1966.

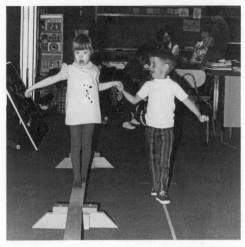

In order to learn, one must have good total body control. Courtesy of the Richardson, Texas Public Schools.

Kraus, there are slightly over six million retarded persons in America today, and approximately three out of every hundred Americans are retarded to some degree.[2] This is a number equivalent to over 3 percent of our total national population. Until recently very little has been done to gain insight into the physical status of the educationally subnormal child and to implement sound physical education programs designed to meet his needs. The reasons for this are varied, ranging from indifference, to fear, to lack of adequate facilities and financing. The potential for helping the mentally retarded child become, through physical activity, a contributing member of society rather than a constant drain on the tax rolls, is great. Community, institutional, teacher-preparation, and research programs are now under way which are concerned with the education of the mentally deficient child.

1. *Community Programs.* There are few community recreation departments in the United States that have a comprehensive program for the retarded that approaches the quality of the programs offered to individuals with merely physical limitations. This is changing, however, thanks to help from the Joseph Kennedy Foundation, the AAHPER, and the federal government. The work has only begun, but there are encouraging signs that community recreation programs for the retarded are increasing in quality and quantity.

2. *Institutional Programs.* Most public institutions for the mentally retarded claim to have a physical education or recreation program, but more often than not, these programs are staffed by poorly trained, underpaid, overworked staff members or part-time employees who must substitute enthusiasm and dedication for professional knowledge of scientifically based physical activity programs. It is safe to say that few, if any,

---

2 Richard Kraus, *Therapeutic Recreation Service* (Philadelphia: W. B. Saunders, 1973), p. 95.

public institutions in the United States have a well-organized physical education program that is integrated into the total school curriculum of the child, and is designed to serve as an integral part of his education.

3. *Teacher Preparation.* Until recently, colleges and universities have been negligent in the preparation of physical educators for work with the mentally retarded. As a result, there is often an undisguised fear of these children, considerable reluctance in involving them in the physical education curriculum, and a general lack of knowledge of appropriate movement experiences and teaching approaches.

4. *Research.* Little research has been done in the area of the physical abilities of the retarded child and the contribution of physical education to his physical and cognitive functioning. Surprisingly little in the way of "hard data" is available to support the belief that physical education and recreation programs are important and can be of benefit to the total functioning of the retarded child. Sound research is the key to more adequate institutional and teacher-preparation programs. Such research evidence will serve as a foundation for more comprehensive physical education and recreation programs for the retarded child.

Characteristics of Retardation

CAUSES

Mental retardation is a condition characterized by faulty development of intelligence which impairs the individual's ability to learn and to adapt to the demands of society. The causes of mental retardation may be classified as:

1. *Organic*—May happen before, during, or after birth or be caused by accident, diseases, or damaging toxic conditions.
2. *Genetic*—May be inherited from one or both parents' genetic deviations. The most common diagnosed forms are classified as (a) mongolism (known as Downs Syndrome), (b) phenylketonuria (PKU), and (c) familial retardation.
3. *Cultural*—Caused by malnutrition of the mother during the prenatal period or of the child after birth, as well as by deprived environmental conditions due to poverty and other socioeconomic causes.

CLASSIFICATION

Children with low intelligence have been classified in a variety of ways. Educators use the rate of learning that the child is capable of or the degree of the defect in terms of his IQ. The following categories are those used most frequently by educators:

1. *The slow learner* (70–90 IQ). The slow learner is mildly retarded and can achieve learning success but requires more time to achieve than does the average child. This condition may be caused by a perceptual-motor disability, cultural deprivation, emotional disturbance, or lack of proper motivation.

2. *The educable* (52–67 IQ). This group is classified as being moderately retarded. They can, with patient assistance, achieve minimal educational success and can learn personal hygiene habits and even gain employment at home or in a sheltered workshop, depending largely upon the degree of skill and intelligence required for securing and keeping a job. Although the majority can function reasonably well in their own neighborhoods, only a few can do so successfully in the total community.

3. *The custodial* (20–35 IQ). Those in this category are severely retarded and subnormal. They require constant supervision throughout life. Some, with patient help and love, can learn a few self-help skills.

4. *The totally dependent* (Under 20 IQ). Often called "human vegetables," those in this group are almost totally helpless and must depend upon others in order to live.

Physical Skills

Those who are mentally retarded are often also physically retarded and score poorly on tests for physical fitness, motor ability, and physical coordination. Some do well, however, in some sports and physical activities including boxing, track and field events, football, tumbling, and simple games. Often those who are behind the normal in skill mastery have led sheltered lives and have not had an opportunity for activity. Many could learn to do and enjoy sports and games but greatly need to be patiently taught the basic movement skills for doing so.

Physical educators and recreation leaders can do much to help the retarded catch up with their normal peers in skill mastery by providing them with a well-planned graded program of activities which gradually increase in complexity and require greater coordinated movement accuracy. Thus, simple games and skills, when mastered, should be replaced by others which are more fun, challenging, and satisfying to do. Although the retarded child or adult will require much more help, praise, and other motivational encouragement than the normal, the leader will be rewarded, just as much as the learner, when the latter can say with glee, "I did it! I did it!" when he does learn to hit or kick a ball after many failures to do so, or to jump the rope, etc.

Teaching Suggestions

Most retarded children have psychomotor, perceptual, and sensory difficulties as well as extremely poor motor coordination. Retarded children can learn an amazing number of physical activities from a teacher with great patience who shows them much loving care and understanding. There are several things it will be helpful for the teacher to keep in mind.

1. Stress large-motor movement activities involving locomotion, manipulation, and stability movements.

2. Know each child's name and be sure that he or she knows yours.

3. "Show" more, explain less.
4. Keep instruction slow, progressive, and brief.
5. Keep rules simple.
6. Provide for many kinds of rhythmical activities.
7. Stress the "fun" element in play.
8. Remember that some children may need manual assistance through certain activities.
9. Include outdoor and camping activities in the program whenever possible.
10. Reduce each skill to its simplest component so that the child can cope with it.
11. Name the movement or skill being taught to help develop vocabulary.
12. Keep practice periods short, with frequent changes in activities in order to reduce frustration.
13. When the child experiences success, let him repeat it several times and enjoy his feeling of accomplishment.
14. Reward accomplishments, no matter how small, with praise.
15. Keep each child active.
16. Set standards of acceptable behavior by praising good performance.
17. Introduce new activities early in the lesson because of the learner's inability to cope with learning new things rapidly.
18. Stress the development of fundamental movement patterns and general movement skills.
19. Whenever possible, include the retarded child in the normal class.

Recreational Programs

It is only recently that public and voluntary agencies have provided recreational programs for the retarded. Formerly, the only programs serving this need were those in custodial institutions, special schools, or private homes. Now such organizations as the National Association for Retarded Children, the American Association for Mental Deficiency, the Department of Health, Education and Welfare, the Kennedy Foundation, and the American Alliance for Health, Physical Education and Recreation are currently sponsoring educational and recreational programs for retardates of all ages.

Recreational programs help retardates learn to use their time more constructively, to increase their social and communicative skills, and to stimulate their physical growth and control of their own bodies—all of which can lead to an early independence from their families, which, in turn, can help them become more successful at school or work.

Because the retarded do not often take part in after-school programs of intramural sports and/or athletics, the community recreation center must make a greater effort to include sports and games, aquatics, and conditioning and self-testing activities in their programs. It is important that they be provided opportunities to have social contacts with the non-disabled as much as possible. Good recreational programs should help the retarded to overcome their frustrations and feelings of uselessness. Such programs can do much also to stimulate their mental development.

The recreation program should provide the mentally retarded with additional opportunities to learn, review and practice many kinds of simple physical play skills. Children especially enjoy improving body control through such activities as jumping, skipping, hopping, swimming, skating, horseback riding, and simple singing games and dances.

The retarded often lack self-confidence because of their many failures, so it is imperative that all educational and recreational programs for them be planned around the things they *can* accomplish. Physical education and recreation programs give the retarded child and adult a chance to come into close contact with people in a fun activity, to cooperate, to learn the necessity of rules and obedience to them, and to develop friendships. Since most of them are social outcasts among their normal peers, the latter is especially valuable.

Leaders in education and recreation, aided by volunteers, should work to interest civic, fraternal, religious and other professional groups in providing educational and recreational program opportunities for the retarded of all ages. As the late John F. Kennedy has said, "Although these individuals may be the victims of Fate, they must not be the victims of our neglect."

SUGGESTED READINGS

BOGARDUS, LADONNA, *Camping with Retarded Persons*. Nashville, Tenn.: Cokesbury, 1970.

CARLSON, BERNICE WELLS, and DAVID GINGLEND, *Recreation for Retarded Teen Agers and Young Adults*. Nashville, Tenn.: Abingdon Press, 1968.

CRATTY, BRYANT J., *Developmental Games for Physically Handicapped Children* (movement activities for neurotically handicapped and retarded children and youth). Palo Alto, Cal.: Peek Publications, 1969.

———, *Developmental Sequences of Perceptual-Motor Tasks*. 1937 Grand Avenue, Baldwin, N.Y.: Educational Activities, Inc., 1967.

———, *Learning and Playing: Fifty Vigorous Activities for the Atypical Child*. Freeport, N.Y.: Educational Activities, 1969.

———, *Motor Activity and the Education of Retardates*. Philadelphia: Lea & Febiger, 1969.

GODFREY, BARBARA B., and NEWELL C. KEPHART, *Movement Patterns and Motor Education*. New York: Appleton-Century-Crofts, 1968.

HJELTE, GEORGE, and JAY SHIVERS, *Public Administration of Recreation Services*. Philadelphia: Lea & Febiger, 1972.

MITCHELL, HELENE JO, and WILLIAM HELLMAN, JR., "The Municipal Recreation Department and Recreation Services for the Mentally Retarded," *Therapeutic Recreation Journal*, 4th Quarter, 1969.

National Easter Seal Society for Crippled Children and Adults, "Rehabilitating the Retarded," *Rehabilitation Literature,* 31, No. 12 (December 1970).

RAMBUSCH, NANCY M., *Learning How to Learn: An American Approach to Montessori.* Baltimore, Md.: Helicern Press, 1962.

STEVENS, ARDIS, *Fun is Therapeutic: A Recreation Book to Help Therapeutic Recreation Leaders by People Who Are Leading Recreation.* Springfield, Ill.: Charles Thomas, 1972.

4

Cerebral Palsy

Cerebral palsy victims have suffered damage to motor control centers of the brain as a result of a disease, anomoly, or accident before, during, or after birth. Cerebral palsy results in a motor disability that may affect many parts of the body or only a limited group of muscles anywhere in the body. It can cause weakness, lack of coordination, involuntary motions, paralysis, drooling, facial grimaces, and excessive rigidity or body stiffness, depending upon the severity and location of brain damage.

Characteristics

In addition to their muscular handicaps, the cerebral palsied usually have multiple handicaps. Many are also retarded, have hearing and vision loss, are emotionally disturbed, and are social outcasts because of their appearance and behavior. It is generally believed that most cerebral palsy victims are lower in intellectual ability than the "normal" population, although many have normal and superior intelligence.[1] It is not surprising that many have an excessive need for affection and independence. Although some victims appear docile and submissive, these feelings often hide underlying hostility and inward rebellion. Many have marked feelings of inferiority and escape reality through excessive daydreaming.

---

[1] Richard Kraus, *Therapeutic Recreation* (Philadelphia: W. B. Saunders, 1973), p. 120.

There is no cure for this disease, for once brain cells are damaged they remain permanently so. Each person should be carefully evaluated by medical and special education experts. Remedial physical and school programs should be geared to build functional developmental patterns for the operative parts of the body that remain. Braces, drugs, surgery, and rehabilitation and physical therapy are used as treatment.

The cerebral palsied, like all handicapped, must learn to live in a society that is mostly normal. Throughout the nation there are sheltered workshops in which those with vocational training can work for various manufacturing companies. The work often requires dull, monotonous movements which normal persons would find boring; however, such repetitious work is well suited for many cerebral palsy victims (as well as other disabled people) and enables them to be financially self-supporting.

CAUSES

Approximately 30 percent of the cases are a result of failure of the brain to develop properly, an infection of the mother during early pregnancy (usually German measles during the first three months), sometimes syphilis, fetal anoxia, cerebral hemorrhage during the fetal stage, the RH blood factor, and other causes of severe metabolic disturbances of the mother.

The majority of cases (60 percent) occur *during* birth. If birth is too rapid, the tiny brain cells may explode, causing brain damage. If it is too slow, anoxia or lack of oxygen may also destroy the brain cells. Head injury resulting in cerebral hemorrhage is another cause. (Contrary to popular belief, only a small percentage of cases result from the faulty use of forceps.) Premature babies are often victims because the weakness of the tiny blood vessels in their brains results in hemorrhage. Vitamin K deficiency in the infant is thought to be another causative factor of this malady.

Only 10 percent of cerebral palsy cases have been caused by head injuries following birth. These may involve accidents, combat in war, infection in the central nervous system from such diseases as meningitis, or from a brain abscess or tumor. A lack of oxygen to the brain as a result of, for example, gas poisoning or choking can also cause CP.

CLASSIFICATION

The five different types of this malady are described below:

The Spastics. Stiffness and limited voluntary control of movement resulting from contracted hypertonic muscles are the chief characteristics of this type. The muscles of the arms and legs contract rapidly when passively stretched. Often the legs are rotated inward, flexed at the hip, with knees adducted. The arms are stiff, elbows flexed, and the lower arms, and fingers are pronated. Body movements are jerky and uncertain.

The spastic person is usually introverted, extremely sensitive and fearful of new situations, tense, and awkward. This type of cerebral palsy is the most prevalent; its victims are often mentally retarded.

The Athetoids. This is the second most common type. Its victims have almost constant involuntary jerky, purposeless movements. When injury of the basal ganglia of the brain (which sort out and permit desired movements to occur) is great, control of speech as well as of the hands and swallowing is minimal. Often a movement starts where a person wants it to but ends up at a different place than intended. These movements vary from very fast to extremely slow responses. Frequently the toes turn back, feet rotate inwardly, and the head is thrown back with the mouth open and drooling. Facial grimaces are common.

The Ataxics. A disturbed sense of balance, direction, and coordination characterizes this group. Ataxics tend to walk in circles, are wobbly, and standing upright or still is a real problem. They are also awkward and have many characteristics of the athetoid. Since kinesthetic awareness is lacking in this group, it is difficult for ataxics to see in three-dimensional space; frequently the eyeballs are involved in rapid, involuntary movements. Although the ataxia victim can understand the basic concepts of reach, grasp, and release, he cannot perform these movements accurately. When he throws a ball, it will go sideways instead of straight; he often spills his food and has much difficulty doing two-handed tasks such as lacing shoes or buttoning. He cannot do school work or other work in a poorly lighted place. Ataxics make up 5 to 10 percent of all cerebral palsy cases.

The Rigidity Group. Mental retardation is also often prevalent in this group, which is characterized by extreme body stiffness or rigidity and the lack of the stretch reflexes. This type is the result of a diffuse rather than a localized brain hemorrhage and is often caused by encephalitis. Often normal movements suddenly are replaced by jerky ones (intermittent rigidity) and resistance to passive movements may often be continuous.

The Tremor Group. In this type of cerebral palsy, tremors appear as uncontrollable movements, and their speed is constant. The tremors are often mixed with muscle rigidity. However, body movements are usually superior to those made by people in the other four palsied groups, and the learning of new movement skills is not such a gigantic struggle. As is true in all types of cerebral palsy cases, however, victims are often in both a social and emotional dilemma—too often they live in a world of social isolation. This group makes up about 5 percent of the total of cerebral palsy cases.

The following terms are also used for classifying the cerebral palsied:

Degrees of Severity

1. *Mild*—ambulatory, understandable speech, use of arms and legs satisfactory

2. *Moderate*—partially disabled, has difficulty moving, speaking, and performing tasks of daily living
3. *Severe*—involvement complete, confined to bed or wheelchair

Involvement Degree
1. *Monoplegic*—one limb involved
2. *Paraplegic*—both legs only
3. *Hemiplegic*—one leg and arm involved on same side of the body, with the arm often being more so than the leg
4. *Triplegic*—involves both legs and one arm; generally spastic
5. *Quadriplegic*—all four extremities involved; in spastics, the legs the most affected; the arms the most damaged among the tremor and athetoid groups

EDUCATIONAL PROGRAMS

Many cerebral palsied need custodial care and are placed in special schools or hospitals where educational programs are provided for them. Some cannot go to school but are serviced by visiting teachers. Others attend special classes in public schools. Some few attend regular school with children of normal intelligence. Regardless of where the child does go to school, the educational program must be tailored to fit his very special needs. Excessive effort must be made by the teacher to help the child want to learn in an environment that is warm, friendly, yet challenging.

The Physical Education Program

This program should be developmental and closely related to physical therapy. The teacher should be a part of the rehabilitation team, working closely with the parents, physician, classroom teacher, and physical therapist. Specific movement exercises—such as movement of the patient's various body parts by the teacher or therapist, followed by the patient making the same movements on his own—are often used. Learning to walk with crutches or alone through lowered parallel bars is often taught at special schools or treatment centers.

Those with only slight handicaps and movement problems can often be in a class with the normal, although activities should be adapted to their limitations. The fun and peer acceptance that develops through playing games should be stressed. Throwing larger balls, catching bouncing balls instead of thrown ones, kicking stationary rather than moving objects, and activities which require the large muscles rather than intricate movements are best. Square and social dancing for older children and rhythmical games for younger children are highly recommended. Skill perfection is not as important a requirement for this group as is

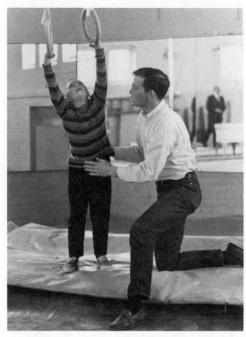

Cerebral-palsied children can learn to do a wide variety of physical activities. Courtesy of the AAHPER.

the gaining of pleasure and the acceptance of others. Swimming is an ideal activity for most, for being in the water is relaxing and allows for greater movement possibilities. Doing exercises to music will prove beneficial, especially since many cerebral palsy victims are obese and/or cannot move their bodies rhythmically. However, because the needs of affected individuals are so different, the program must be uniquely designed for each one. Rest periods should be frequent and students should be taught the various kinds of relaxing techniques.

If the class is composed entirely of cerebral palsied, the teacher must realize that those afflicted, whether they be spastics, athetoids, or ataxics, differ greatly. The spastics can be more successful in activities requiring constant, flowing movements. Among the athetoids, relaxation should be stressed. Balance activities are not suitable for the ataxics. All in the class, however, should be encouraged to develop smoother movement patterns and be taught activities with high carry-over value for later life and for present leisure-time activities.

Suggested activities include:

Archery	Running games and relays
Billiards	Shuffleboard
Bowling	Simple folk and square dances
Camping and outing	Simple games
Croquet	Swimming
Horseshoes	

The Recreation Program

Although the cerebral palsied cannot be cured, victims can be helped through a variety of modalities, including recreation. The primary function of the recreation program should be to stimulate physical and intellectual growth and to help each participant gain needed physical and social skills so that each can, in turn, become more acceptable as a member of a normal group of peers. Because those afflicted by this handicap are classified as mild, moderate, or severe, the amount of progress each person makes toward the attainment of needed skills depends upon how much brain damage is involved, coupled with the degree of motivation to work around unchangeable limitations. Consequently, it is imperative that the recreation leader, like the school teacher and physical education specialist, know as much about each individual in the group as possible. This means that information must be gathered about the extent of the physical damage, the patient's home and family life, present limitations, attitudes toward himself and his place in society, present recreational pursuits, and other pertinent information.

The resulting recreation program, established on the findings of such information, should be one that does not require quick-action response (such as trying to catch thrown balls of varying sizes) or activities that could produce anxiety (such as highly competitive events). Again, swimming is an ideal recreational activity, especially so for the spastics and those in the rigidity group.

Other recommended activities include arts and crafts, social events such as birthday parties, table games including bridge, visitation trips, homemaking projects such as cooking or repairing furniture, and discussion groups. Although social and folk dance are popular with all age groups, both activities are especially good for lonely teenagers, who often are deserted by their normal peer friends who are beginning to date and go to parties. Day and overnight camping, campcraft, and nature activities are popular with all age groups.

It is imperative that those taking part in the program be involved in planning and carrying it out. The recreation leader should function primarily as a coordinator and resource person who focuses on helping each handicapped person to take part in the program and gain, through this participation, more independence, self-confidence, and happiness.

SUGGESTED READINGS

CRUICKSHANK, W. M., *Cerebral Palsy, Its Individual and Community Problems.* Syracuse: Syracuse University Press, 1966.

DENHOFF, E., and I. ROBINAULT, *Cerebral Palsy and Related Disorders.* New York: McGraw-Hill, 1960.

FRIEBURG, W. H., and GAROLD EALIN, *Recreation for the Handicapped*. Carbondale, Ill.: Southern Illinois University Press, 1965.

KEPHART, N. C., *The Slow Learner in the Classroom*. Columbus, Ohio: Charles G. Merrill Co., 1960.

National Easter Seal Society for Crippled Children and Adults, "Cerebral Palsy Viewed by Its Victim," *Rehabilitation Literature*, 3, No. 11 (November 1970).

ROBINS, FERRIS, *Educational Rhythmics for Mentally and Physically Handicapped Children*. New York: Association Press, 1968.

Swimming for the Cerebral Palsied. United Cerebral Palsy Association, 66 East 34th Street, New York 10016, 1958.

TOWBIN, ARTHUR, *The Pathology of Cerebral Palsy*. Springfield, Ill.: Charles Thomas, 1960.

WHEELER, HELEN, and AGNES HOOLEY, *Physical Education for the Handicapped*. Philadelphia: Lea & Febiger, 1969.

Publications from the United Cerebral Palsy Association, 66 E. 34th St., New York, 10016

More Than Fun, a handbook of Recreational Programming for Children and Adults with Cerebral Palsy.

Recreation for the Homebound Person with Cerebral Palsy.

5

Visual and Auditory Handicaps

VISUAL HANDICAPS

There are many kinds of vision problems as well as degrees of blindness. Uncorrected faulty vision can cause deep-seated learning, emotional, and physical problems. Hyperopia, (farsightedness) and myopia (nearsightedness), and color-blindness, strabismus or muscular imbalance (which results in a cross-eyed condition or marked facial squint) are all common problems among thousands of children and adults in our society.

Visual acuity is most often measured in schools by the Snellen Eye Chart Test, in which the letters on each line of the chart are smaller than those of the line above. Normal vision is 20/20, meaning that a person can read the letters of the line marked for 20 feet. The E test is also often used for preschoolers and others. For this, the person being tested points his fingers or hand the way the legs of the letter E point. Because most of our learning comes through our eyes and ears, it is vitally important that all children have their vision and hearing checked and corrected by the age of four, and that those with problems have them treated before starting to school. Today it has been estimated that there are over 18,000 children who must read Braille or large-type books to gain their education.[1]

---

[1] Charles Buell, *Physical Education for Blind Children* (Springfield, Ill.: Charles Thomas, 1966), p. 3.

Blindness at birth is far more handicapping than that which occurs later in life, for it prevents the person from understanding visual symbols and such concepts as big-little, near-far, beautiful-ugly, clean-dirty, etc.

Characteristics

The blind tend to be obese due to lack of large-muscle activities such as running, jumping, and skipping. Many have poor posture and coordination. Peculiar mannerisms known as *blindisms* are common, especially among children. Examples are rocking back and forth, frequent eye rubbing with the fists, turning around and around like a spinning top, hand waving in front of the face, and head nodding. Among both the blind and the partially sighted are often found individuals who tend to be:

1. Educationally retarded in comparison to normal individuals
2. Awkward when moving through space and poor at activities that call for the coordinated movements of the small muscles of the body
3. Socially immature and ill at ease, especially when meeting strangers or in new social situations
4. Lower in intelligence than the normal
5. More likely to have emotional and personality problems
6. Afraid to try to master new things, especially new kinds of physical activities
7. Sedentary, solitary, and engaged in fantasies and daydreams
8. Often depressed, and feel rejected by parents, family, and normal peers
9. Keener of hearing, feeling, tasting, and smelling than the normal, with a more marked kinesthetic sense so that they avoid running into walls or stumbling over curbs (referred to as *obstacle perception*)
10. Reluctant to take part in activities that require speed, strength, skill, and physical endurance
11. Fearful of the future with its lack of opportunities for marriage and/or parenthood
12. Overprotected by parents, smothered by too much attention and guilt-centered parental "love"

CAUSES

Blindness can be caused by accidents, diseases such as trachoma, ophthalmia, or gonorrhea (which leads to prenatal blindness), and heredity. Scarlet fever, typhoid fever, smallpox, and measles can also result in serious eye defects. Accidents, the chief cause of death among elementary school children, often cause total or partial blindness.

It has been estimated that there are over a quarter million blind people (including children) in the United States, and there are twice as many who are only partially sighted.[2] As Wheeler and Hooley point out,

---

[2] Arthur Daniels and Evelyn Davies, *Adapted Physical Education*, 2nd ed. (New York: Harper & Row, 1965), p. 261.

partially seeing and blind children share the following common characteristics:

1. They favor solitary pursuits which permit them to start and stop and move about in space as they will. Such activities as they choose protect them from injury and from the failure which might result from competition with others, yet provide them with the satisfaction of having moved. Often their choice is sedentary activities in contrast with the more active occupations chosen by the normal child. Seldom do they participate in activities which lead to strength, speed, and endurance.
2. They may display symptoms of fear, frustration, concern over the future, worry about social maturity, especially with regard to the opposite sex.[3]

DEFINITIONS

The *blind* person has a vision acuity of 20/200 or less. Such an individual may be totally blind in both eyes or in one or barely able to distinguish motion or light. Blind children are usually enrolled in special schools for the blind.

The *partially sighted* person has visual acuity ranging from 20/70 to 20/200 and can see some light, forms, a few bright colors as well as black and white, and can detect some movements. He may be enrolled in a special or regular school, depending upon the degree of his visual defect. Increasingly today, those who are partially sighted attend regular schools wherein they have specialized instruction in the communicative arts and attend certain other classes with normal children.

Internal strabismus is a type of muscular imbalance which causes the eyes to turn inward. *External strabismus* causes the eyes to turn outward. *Alternating strabimus* causes the eyes to turn inward and then outward. *Hyperphoria* causes the eyes to turn upward or downward. All these defects can usually be corrected by an *ophthalmologist,* who is a licensed physician. (An *optometrist* is a nonmedical practitioner certified to prescribe and fit glasses as well as treat eye defects without surgery or drugs; an *optician* is licensed to grind lenses and fit glasses.) Often an ophthalmologist is assisted by an *orthoptist,* who directs eye exercises as prescribed by a physician.

All children need vigorous physical activity in order to grow and maintain a healthy body. Likewise, all people, regardless of age, need to know how to play, for it is one of the great physical needs of man, along with food, rest, elimination, and sex. All people also need to be able to move successfully through space, to mingle with and be a part of a group, to love and be loved. The handicapped, who have many additional kinds of problems, must learn to accept their limitations and find ways to work around them. At school the primary responsibility of the teacher is to establish and maintain the best kind of learning en-

---

[3] Ruth Wheeler and Agnes Hooley, *Physical Education for the Handicapped* (Philadelphia: Lea & Febiger, 1969), pp. 251–52.

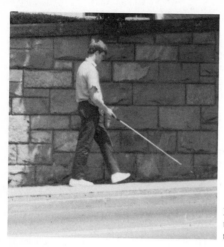

Learning to cane walk is also taking steps toward greater independence. Courtesy of the California School for the Blind.

vironment possible for *all* students so that each one can learn, grow, and develop according to his own unique pattern for self-improvement. Extreme care must be taken when working with the blind and partially sighted to assure that the tasks provided for them are conducted in the safest kind of an environment possible. The teacher-leader must not rob any child of learning experiences by doing things *for* him instead of *with* him or by letting his peers do so.

Vigorous physical activities should be a vital part of the educational program for both the normal and the handicapped. Dr. Charles Buell, a nationally recognized authority on physical activities for the blind, has declared:

> Physical fitness is important for all of us, but particularly for blind individuals. A blind person must expend much more energy to reach the same rung of success as an individual who has normal vision. Regardless of limitations in budget, facilities or physical handicap, we must provide our children, including those who are blind, the daily minimum of vigorous exercise they need for physical development.[4]

Teaching Suggestions

Teaching the visually handicapped requires the possession of the finest kind of instructional skills. Above all, the teacher must have empathy for her students, coupled with much patience, and be keenly interested in helping each person learn desired physical skills. Often the feet and hands of the sightless should be guided by the teacher so that they get the kinesthetic feel of the movement, whether they are learning to throw a softball or kick a soccer ball. This individualized attention, however, should be given in such a way that at the same time the rest

---

[4] Buell, *Physical Education for Blind Children*, p. 5.

of the class is busily engaged in other learning tasks. The teacher must also be skilled in giving brief and accurate verbal communication. Often by blindfolding her own eyes or closing them she can better grasp the complications involved in learning various movements. Some helpful teaching hints follow:

1. Use a whistle when wanting the class to move or stop.
2. Use a turning point for outdoor races that will guide the feet of the runners. Mats should be used for this purpose for indoor races or relays.
3. Clearly mark field dimensions and safety hazards in bright colors.
4. Use a bell or whistle ahead of the ball in order to help the players know where it is on the field in team games.
5. Have the students read game rules and other information in Braille before actually playing a game.
6. Use many auditory cues to help the student gain a quicker understanding of space and distances.
7. Use sighted assistants. (Teenagers are especially fine helpers, for they often are strongly motivated to be of service and tend to be more objective about the handicapped than are adults.)
8. Set definite goals with and for student, and objectives to be reached.
9. Use music often both for relaxation and motivation.
10. Include as many strenuous big-muscle activities as possible.

Almost all the activities suitable for normal children can be modified for use with the handicapped. Free play times as well as individual

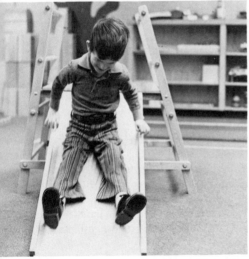

Partially sighted children, as well as those who are totally blind, can learn many physical activities, including this one. Courtesy of the Richardson, Texas Public Schools.

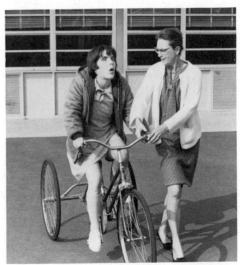

Learning to ride a bicycle can be a great adventure! Courtesy of the Los Angeles Public Schools.

instruction should be given to these children. Above all, the class should not number more than fifteen students—less if there are many who need special help. Generally speaking, homogeneous skill grouping is best rather than age or sex grouping. Because many of the students lag far behind normal children of the same chronological age, games and activities suited for much younger children can be used. The teacher must accept the child where he or she actually *is* in relation to skill mastery and then help that child advance to a higher level of achievement.

SPECIAL EQUIPMENT

Balls used by the blind should have bells or rattles inside them and be painted yellow or white; they should also be larger and softer than those used by normal children. The play area for children should contain jungle gyms, turning bars, monkey ladders, swings, teeter-totters, and sand boxes. The play area should be fence-enclosed and relatively free of natural hazards. Guide wires which runners can grasp should be used for track events, for they will enable the students to run freely at top speed. These can easily be made by stretching wires above head level over the running area and attaching short ropes with metal rings on the other end. The runner holds a pair of rings to enable him to move quickly in safe lines as the ropes slide along the wires.[5]

Other suggested equipment aids to teaching the blind include:

- Swimming—inflated swim trainer belts, which leave the instructor's hands free to assist the student
- Softball—base paths in dirt, or raised cement for contrast
- Trampoline—a bell under the center for placement and some type of a sounding device at the end of the trampoline for direction
- Basketball—metronomes on the backboard for shooting direction; orange-colored circle in center for partially sighted
- General exercises—activity records for smaller children to make activities more interesting

An audible goal locator is available from the American Printing House for the Blind in Louisville, Kentucky. Gym scooters can be made by putting four casters and wheels on boards. A portable aluminum bowling rail can be purchased from the American Foundation for the Blind in New York City. Many teachers use their ingenuity as well as their knowledge of the particular problems of the blind to design equipment for students to use. Some of the best ideas for usable equipment can come from the students themselves and their parents.

---

[5] See the excellent colored film of the many kinds of physical activities and equipment for the blind, *Recreation for the Blind*, available for rental from Dr. Charles Buell, California School for The Blind, 3001 Derby Street, Berkeley, California. Also available from this source are *Recreation for the Blind*, and *Motor Performance of Visually Handicapped Children*.

The Physical Education and Recreation Program

Activities that are best suited for instruction of the blind and partially sighted in physical education include:

Dance

Folk	Social
Square	Tap
Modern	Movement exploration

Individual Activities

Bag punching	Physical fitness testing
Camping and hiking	Rope jumping
Fly and bait casting	Rowing
Baseball	Swimming and diving
Basketball	Shuffleboard
Billiards	Stunts and tumbling
Bowling	Trampolining
Gymnastics	Volleyball
Horseshoes	Weight lifting
Hiking	Wrestling
Ice and roller skating	

Rope jumping, ice and roller skating, bowling, trampolining, swimming, hiking, dancing, physical fitness testing, and wrestling are the most popular activities.

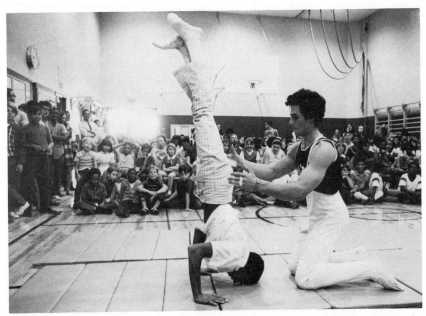

Stunts and tumbling are ideal activities for some handicapped children such as the blind or deaf. Courtesy of the Los Angeles Public Schools.

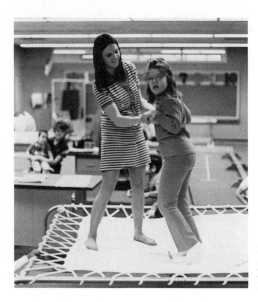

Even though you can't see, a good teacher can help you learn to jump on a trampoline. Courtesy of the Richardson, Texas Public Schools.

Recreational programs for the blind should include all kinds of social activities that will provide fun and fellowship. Parties, guessing games, holiday celebrations, puzzles and tricks, singing games, table games (such as Braille dominoes and cards), dramatics, music, dance, and camping should also have a big place in the program. Many opportunities should be provided for the participants to mix, mingle, and play with their normal peers on both a one-to-one and a group basis.[6]

Scouting is an ideal activity for the visually handicapped child, but only one such child should be in any one group. Churches, the YWCA, and the YMCA also provide splendid recreational outlets for both youngsters and adults. Participation in neighborhood activities seems to be easier for visually handicapped children than for teenagers; often, contact with normal peers is lost when normally sighted boys and girls begin dating.

Many city recreation departments are adding nature trails in parks and wooded areas, marked in Braille for the blind.[7] Trips and excursions are also added to the program, as are hobby and club groups. Camping is an ideal activity for the blind of all ages; there are over sixty camps in America specifically for the blind. In these camps program activities include swimming, crafts, hiking, boating, fishing, horseback riding, and campcraft activities.

The Speed Museum in Louisville, Kentucky, is one of the many museums that have developed an art program for blind children. Objects

---

[6] For directions in teaching these activities, see Maryhelen Vannier, *Recreation Leadership*, 3rd ed. (Philadelphia: Lea & Febiger, 1975).

[7] See the interesting article by Joseph Gowey, "Touch and See," in the November 1969 issue of *Parks and Recreation Journal* for directions to lay out nature trails and program possibilities for the blind.

on display at these museums are those children can touch, such as fine wood carvings, statues of people and/or animals, and objects made from yarn, plastic, or other tactile materials.

Far more special schools than public ones provide opportunities for after-school sport competition for the blind or partially sighted. Teams may be made up of all visually handicapped players or they may be mixed, with only one or two being atypical and the rest normal. Wrestling is by far the most widely used competitive sport. Other popular activities are swimming, track and field, bowling, and gymnastics. In public schools the competitive activities included in most programs are softball, football, basketball, and track and field; these sports are better suited to the partially sighted than to the blind.

AUDITORY HANDICAPS

Hearing difficulty is one of the most common defects found in children and adults, and hearing loss ranges from partial to complete. Many children are mistakenly labeled as retarded or slow learners when their learning problem is actually caused by deafness.

The *hard of hearing* can hear enough to learn how to speak and may or may not wear a hearing aid. Those classified as *deaf* (from birth) cannot hear nor speak unless taught to do so by a speech specialist. *Hearing acuity* is measured in tone or pitch and *intensity* by decibels. All school children should be given a screen hearing test annually and the tester should be a trained audiometry technician.

Types of screen tests include the sweep check audiometer test and the Massachusetts pure-tone test. Those with hearing loss should be given a more complete examination by an otologist, who can trace the source of hearing loss in order to determine if the defect is caused by excessive ear wax, involvement in the inner ear, or improper sensorineural development. Because speech and language are vital in our society, every effort should be made to correct defects as early as possible. It has been estimated that at least 5 percent of all school-age children have serious hearing problems, that there are approximately 760,000 youth and adults who are totally deaf, and that hearing loss is on a rapid increase throughout the nation, especially in metropolitan areas.

Characteristics

Various types of hearing impairments include:

1. *Psychogenic deafness*—associated with mental illness and emotional disturbance and not physiologically caused
2. *Central deafness*—caused by diseases of the brain such as tumor, arteriosclerosis, cerebral hemorrhage, or multiple sclerosis
3. *Sensorineural impairment*—due to prenatal factors (the RH factor and infections such as measles and flu in the first three months of pregnancy);

natal causes (meningitis, measles, mumps, head injuries, acoustic trauma); and postnatal causes (tumor, degenerative diseases, accidents)

4. *Conductive loss*—caused by impairments in the outer or middle ear or the Eustachian tubes

5. *Congenital deafness*—caused by nerve injury during birth or an inherited defect

It is important that all persons having hearing defects receive help. Children should have assistance as early as possible and be well placed in either a special school for the deaf or in a regular school where speech or reading specialists teach deaf students how to communicate with others.

The following may be signs of hearing impairment:

1. Faulty speech patterns; faulty pitch, tone, or volume
2. Holding the head to one side, inattentiveness, excessive daydreaming, inability to follow directions
3. Inability to detect who is speaking and what is being said
4. Emotional instability; hostility or extreme withdrawal
5. Failure in school
6. Difficulty in maintaining balance
7. Inability to join class discussions and group games
8. Social inferiority

Those who are diagnosed as having nerve deafness (markedly severe or complete deafness) should be placed in schools for the deaf, for this type of disability is incurable and prohibits the successful use of hearing aids. The deaf and those who are hard of hearing respond better if they are separated in school for instructional purposes. In most cases the teacher will need medical assistance if a deaf child is to be placed in a class with normal children. Special teachers are needed to instruct the child in lip-reading and speaking.

Most deaf persons are behind their normal peers educationally, physically, and socially. Those with partial hearing tend to be more stable, more outgoing, and more socially sure than the totally deaf. They also tend to talk loudly and a lot as well as using excessive facial gestures and rapid hand movements. Many deaf people are shy, sedentary isolates. Often they are obese and many lack good physical skills, balance, and coordination. There is a great variation among the deaf; some can lip-read and talk; others are totally mute and seemingly in a daze. All need assistance in developing communicative skills. All also need to learn to heed warning danger signals for their own survival.

Teaching Suggestions

It is possible for a teacher who is skilled in teaching the normal to learn to become a master physical educator for the deaf, assuming he or she has (1) a willingness to experiment in order to develop the best methods of communicating and teaching and (2) the ability to profit from failures.

It is important for the teacher-leader to be visible to all members of the class. Colorful visual aids are relied on heavily in teaching the deaf. Above all, class groups should be kept small; rapport must be quickly established between the teacher and learner; and every student must be given an abundance of approval, affection, and a sense of achievement. Mastery of these three A's are basic to success for any educator, but especially to those working with the handicapped.

The Physical Education and Recreation Program

Many of the deaf and partially hearing students can be successfully placed in a regular physical education class or a modified one in which there are students with other kinds of handicaps. However, this can only be successful if the teacher realizes the seriousness of problems of communication each person has; skill in teaching through clear demonstration as well as verbal instructions is necessary. The key decision concerns which type of class would best meet the needs and interests of the student and the class as a whole. Those who have severe or recent hearing loss can profit most from an individualized program for a small homogeneous group of not more than eight to ten.

Many of the hard of hearing wear hearing aids, and most of them are afraid to run, jump, skip, or hop for fear of damaging this device. Difficulty in hearing instructions may cause rude or disinterested behavior by the hard of hearing. To avoid this, all game and safety rules should be made clear before the instruction and/or free-play periods begin. Deaf students usually need more factual knowledge concerning sports and games than do the normal; these can often best be understood through a liberal use of visual aids such as movies, slides, posters, and charts.

Ideal class size for groups of the totally deaf is ten. Clear-cut class beginning and ending cues are needed. All the students should be arranged in fan formation for instructional purposes rather than in a single formation, so that all can see the teacher.

YOUNG CHILDREN

A wide range of activities should be taught to young children. These include simple and creative games such as Red Rover and games the children make up, leadup games to sports such as Newcomb for volleyball,[8] Kickball for softball, and Twenty-one for basketball. Because deaf children, like most other handicapped persons, tend to be obese, they may lack body coordination and the ability to balance when moving through space. Thus, a physical activity program can be of great value to this group. The program should also include activities in movement exploration in which the child may be led into activity by such ques-

---

[8] In this game, the ball is caught and then thrown back across the net instead of being hit over it.

tions as "Who can run in the fastest circle?" or "If you were a pony, how would you gallop?" Graded stunts and tumbling, as well as elementary gymnastic activities, should be part of the program. Cartwheels, headstands, walking on a low balance beam, and the duck walk are some activities that can be taught. Track and field events that call for much running and jumping are especially ideal for those children not wearing hearing aids, to help build endurance and other fitness aspects quickly. Aquatic activities such as elementary swimming and boating and canoeing should be included in the program. Provisions should be made for the children to take part in supervised free-play periods, to play on a one-to-one basis as well as in groups or teams.

OLDER YOUTH AND ADULTS

A wide variety of physical fitness exercises and tests should be basic to the program for these age groups. Boys and men will respond well to body-building classes, girls to those in figure and weight control. Dance (social, modern, and folk) has a great appeal; music can play an important role in developing finer coordination for those who are not totally deaf. Track and field events, aquatics, and many kinds of individual sports such as fencing, golf, or archery and many kinds of team activities such as field hockey or basketball should also be included in the program. Many deaf students can play basketball, especially, with amazing skill, for they can see well and stop on the referee's whistle, the vibrations of which they can feel through their feet. Actually, almost any activity the normal sighted person can do is a good physical activity choice for the deaf. Learning to play a lifetime sport well, such as tennis or golf, will not only lead to active participation in later life during leisure time but also give a student increased opportunity for making social contacts through gaining skill in a popular sport.

Almost all the activities that have been suggested for the visually handicapped can also be used successfully for those with hearing problems. Camping and gardening will bring fun to many, as will photography, painting, and learning to make beautiful things with one's own hands. Musical activities are less appealing to this handicapped group and should not be stressed as much as are art, drama, or vigorous physical activities. Because many deaf people have posture and movement problems, body mechanics, physical fitness, and posture correction should play a role in the total program offerings.

Like the blind, many deaf people thrive upon competition. Most of them can play on teams in basketball, football, and baseball remarkably well. Many become expert in individual sports such as bowling, swimming, or weight lifting. All those interested in joining competitive teams or competing as an individual should be encouraged to do so. Boxing, golf, and high diving should not be included in the program because of the danger of head and/or ear injury. Those who suffer from ringing in the ears (known medically as tinnitus) should never compete in a noisy facility. Those who have severe problems of balance should not be exposed to or compete in activities that require good balance (such as certain kinds of gymnastic stunts or trampolining).

SUGGESTED READINGS

In Braille, *Physical Education for High School Students*. Washington, D.C., AAHPER, 1972.

BELENKY, ROBERT, *Swimming Program for Blind Children*. New York: American Foundation for the Blind, 1955.

BUELL, CHARLES, *Active Games for the Blind*. Ann Arbor: Edwards Brothers, 1953.

————, *Motor Performance of Visually Handicapped Children*. Ann Arbor: Edwards Brothers, 1950.

————, *Sports for the Blind*. New York: American Foundation for the Blind, 1947.

————, *Physical Education for Blind Children*. Springfield, Ill.: Charles Thomas, 1966.

CLARKE, H. H., and D. H. CLARKE, *Developmental and Adapted Physical Education*. Englewood Cliffs, N.J.: Prentice-Hall, 1963.

CRATTY, BRYANT, *Movement Behavior and Motor Learning*. 2nd ed. Philadelphia: Lea & Febiger, 1967.

FRAMPTON, M. C., and G. MITCHELL, *Camping for Blind Youth*. New York: New York Institute for the Blind, 1949.

KIRK, S. R., *Educating Exceptional Children*. Boston: Houghton Mifflin, 1962.

National Easter Seal Society for Crippled Children and Adults, "Achievement Potential and Rehabilitation of the Deaf," *Rehabilitation Literature*, 31, No. 9 (September 1970).

RITTER, CHARLES, *Hobbies of Blind Adults*. New York: American Foundation for the Blind, 1953.

VANNIER, MARYHELEN, MILDRED FOSTER, and DAVID GALLAHUE, *Teaching Physical Education in Elementary Schools*, 5th ed. Philadelphia: W. B. Saunders, 1973.

VANNIER, MARYHELEN, and HOLLIS FAIT, *Teaching Physical Education in Secondary Schools*, 4th ed. Philadelphia: W. B. Saunders, 1975.

6

Orthopedic Handicaps

There are many kinds of orthopedic handicaps, some easily detectable, others not quickly recognized. Some persons are born minus a hand or fingers; some have deformities of the head or trunk; some walk with the aid of crutches; others are pushed or propel themselves in wheelchairs. (Although few crippled people become professional beggars in America, this is a common practice in many countries throughout the world. In some countries crippled children are even rented out to procurers who take them to beg in places where wealthy foreigners tour. In some of these backward nations, poor parents often look upon having a defective offspring as a disguised financial blessing.) Orthopedic disabilities involve varying degrees of seriousness, and the causes are varied. Some are relatively simple to treat, such as round shoulders; some are chronic and debilitating, such as certain types of arthritis; still others are permanent and incurable, such as spinal bifida. In this chapter we include in the category of orthopedic disabilities any defects that involve bones, joints, and muscles. It is important to recognize that all such ailments can be treated, if not cured, by specific physical exercises; and a physical education and recreation program should be an important part of the lives of those who are so handicapped.

A crippled child is defined as

one, under twenty-one years of age, who by reason of congenital or acquired defects of development, disease or wound, is, or may be expected to become, deficient in use of his body or limbs (an orthopedic cripple) including harelip, cleft palate, and some other handicaps yielding to plastic surgery, and excluding physical difficulties wholly of sight, hearing, or speech, and those affecting the heart primarily, and also excluding serious mental or moral abnormalities unless found in conjunction with orthopedic defects.[1]

The above is a broad definition. However, this chapter is concerned not only with those seriously orthopedically handicapped who are unable to perform body movements properly (walking, running, throwing, etc.) but also with people whose handicaps only slightly limit activities (such as the person with bowlegs). Interest in such persons by the general public is now at an all-time high. Special schools and hospitals have been provided in most states for those most seriously affected. Rehabilitation centers have been established for them, and vocational opportunities are opening to those who qualify for gainful employment. For these victims, as well as for the ones with less serious defects, physical activity is all-important.

The field of therapeutic recreation is increasingly drawing more applicants seeking a career in working with such special groups.

Characteristics and Problems of the Crippled

The emotional problems of people who are limited because of orthopedic handicaps are something to be considered and treated seriously. Neither the crippled child nor the uncoordinated, knock-kneed child can compete with "normal" peers in sports and games. Although some compensate and become recognized as outstanding in their schoolwork or in passive table games such as chess, many develop deep-rooted emotional problems, especially if their parents shelter them too much and there is sibling rivalry in the family.

The age of the person and the suddenness with which any incapacitating disability strikes have a great effect upon the length of time and the type of therapy required for the adjustment that must be made. Those in their teens or older who lose an arm or leg by amputation usually have a more serious adjustment problem to solve than children born with a missing limb or other structural defects. As these persons develop compensatory skills through which they can gain peer and family recognition, they will also gain more stability emotionally. As their newly found activities bring them challenge, increased energy, and more enthusiasm for life, they will also provide positive outlets for hostility and aggression, and thereby aid in the achievement of well-balanced lives.

CAUSES

The main causes of crippling defects are diseases and infections, accidents, congenital birth abnormalities, osteochondrosis, and war. Thou-

---

[1] White House Conference on Child Health and Protection, *The Handicapped Child* (New York: Appleton-Century, 1933), p. 119.

sands of babies are affected by birth defects, many due to contagious diseases such as measles, poliomyelitis, osteomyelitis, and tuberculosis. Dangerous drugs such as LSD and "speed" have been found to cause organic damage to the brain in experimental animals. Experiments in which LSD is applied to human white blood cells indicate that it may cause chromosome breakage, which could result in defective children.[2]

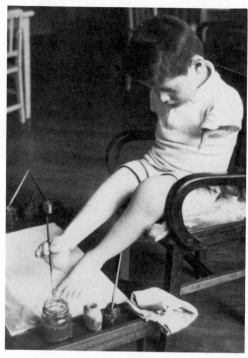

Some children are born defective. Courtesy of Rehabilitation International.

Cancer, if found in the bones of the arms or legs, often leads to amputation of limbs, and it causes crippling defects when found in the spine, joints, or other parts of the body.

Congenital abnormalities and birth deformities such as dislocated, missing, or shortened limbs; club feet; scoliosis; spinal bifida; and wry neck are easily recognizable at birth. Accidents, which are the chief cause of death of children, yearly deform temporarily or permanently millions of Americans of all ages. In the group of those 15 to 24 years old, accidents claim more lives than all other causes combined, including cancer, suicide, homicide, heart disease, and congenital malformations.[3] Because participation in sports and recreation is increasing in our country among all age groups, many players are victims of broken bones, sprains, and

[2] George Lingeman, *Drugs From A to Z* (New York: McGraw-Hill, 1969).

[3] Charles Bucher, Einar Olsen, and Carl Willgoose, *The Foundations of Health* (New York: Appleton-Century-Crofts, 1967), p. 144.

dislocations of a serious nature. Our veteran's hospitals are full of those who have been crippled for life during war actions.

The epidemic of post-rubella anomalies in Australia in 1940 and 1941 and the pandemic of thalidomide embryopathies in Europe in 1960 and 1961 resulted in thousands of births of deformed children. Many were born without arms or legs or had other gross kinds of congenital malformations owing to inborn errors of metabolism caused by drugs taken by the mother during pregnancy. In medical practice only those congenital deformities which are clearly visible at birth or are easily identifiable by X-ray or photographs are recorded on birth certificates. In practice, this policy is not always followed, for although mongolism can be detected at birth, the recording and/or the clinical diagnosis of it is often delayed for several months. Mental retardation, cerebral palsy, blindness, deafness, and epilepsy usually cannot be accurately diagnosed for months following birth or during the early years of childhood. On the other hand, defects like fused fingers, a missing limb, or other gross deformities are obvious. Because it is important that corrective programs begin as early as possible, greater effort must be made to identify deformities or functional defects earlier so that these programs do become a reality.

The Physical Education Program

The physical education program for the orthopedically handicapped should be carefully planned around the specific movement, health, and physical fitness needs of each participant. It may be conducted on an individual or small-group basis with the class composed of all crippled persons, or certain individuals may be placed in a class composed of those with a wide variety of physical handicaps. The leader must have skills in working with this group as well as knowledge about the cause and nature of the disability.

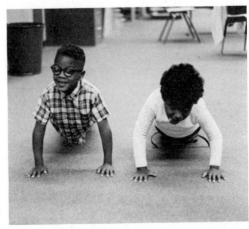

Developing shoulder girdle strength is a must for paraplegics. Courtesy of the Richardson, Texas Public Schools.

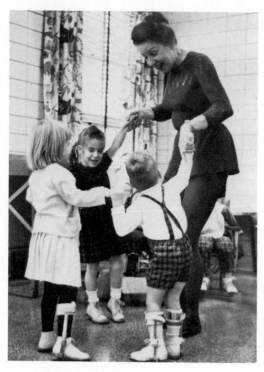

Circle games can help children learn how to move to the left or right as well as how to follow directions. Courtesy of the AAHPER.

The type of activities to be included in the program depends upon the age, kinds of injuries or defects, available facilities, and the specific developmental needs of each participant. The objectives of the program should be to aid each person to (a) develop improved physical fitness, (b) increase total body coordination and movement skills, and (c) learn activities that will lead to a more active and happier life. Therapeutic exercises as well as modified active games and sports, rhythms, dance, and swimming, when appropriate, should constitute the major portion of the program. Medical authorities should aid in planning the program and be asked to prescribe specific developmental exercises for the various individuals in the group. The program should be progressive so that, as a student masters a learning task, a harder one is chosen to challenge him and keep his interest high in constantly improving and learning new skills.

COMPETITIVE SPORTS

Following World War II, wheelchair sports were developed in VA Hospitals all over America as a part of rehabilitation treatment. The first wheelchair basketball tournament was held at the University of Illinois in 1949 and from this event developed the National Wheelchair Basketball Association. The Stokes-Mandeville games held at the Stokes-Mandeville Hospital in Aylesburg, England, in 1947 consisted of competition in archery only. These games soon grew into international competitive events which now include archery, lawn-bowling, table tennis, shotput, javelin, club throw, wheelchair basketball, fencing, snooker, swimming, and weight lifting.

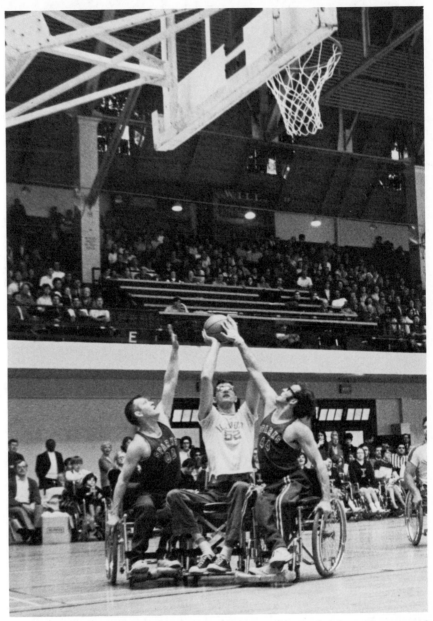

The National Wheelchair Basketball Association is made up of eight conferences and more than fifty teams. Courtesy of the AAHPER.

In 1958 the National Wheelchair Games Committee organized the National Wheelchair Athletic Association to set rules governing wheelchair sports competition in all events mentioned above with the exception of basketball, which had its own governing body. In 1960 United States teams entered international competition in athletic contests for the first time; it was also in this year that the first wheelchair games were

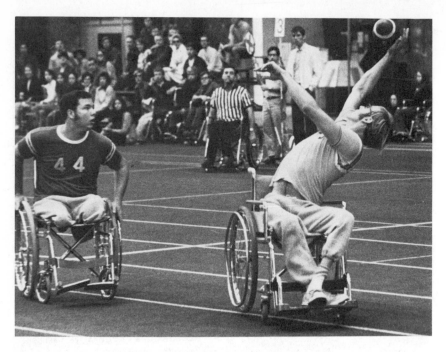

Just because one is confined to a wheelchair does not mean he cannot enjoy team games. Courtesy of the AAHPER.

held in connection with the Olympic games. Disabled athletes from all over the world took part in these events, now known as the Paralympics and held every four years following the Olympic games. The Pan American Council, which has developed from the vast interest in sports competition for paraplegics, now provides wheelchair competition for athletes in the countries of North and South America.

Today over 10,000 disabled men and women American athletes take part in organized competition, and over fifty-six nations throughout the world are a vital part of this international program.[4] Since 1960, United States wheelchair teams have competed in Argentina, Brazil, Canada, Jamaica, Japan, Great Britain, Israel, Italy, France, Hawaii, Hong Kong, Spain, and Ireland. In 1971, international competition was held in Jamaica, and the Paralympics were in Munich, Germany, in 1972, following the Olympic games.

Track competition for wheelchair athletes is held at both the national and international level. Track events include 40-, 60-, and 100-yard dashes; 220- and 440-yard dashes; the 880-yard and mile "run" as distance races; the 240- and 400-yard shuttle relays; and the 880-yard and mile relays. The discus, javelin and precision javelin throw, and the shotput are included in field events. Wheelchair track events are governed by NCAA rules with game modifications.

In 1970, the world's record for the 100-yard dash was 19.1 seconds; that for the mile run was 6.30 seconds; the shotput record was more

[4] Richard Kraus, *Therapeutic Recreation* (Philadelphia: W. B. Saunders, 1973), pp. 129–31.

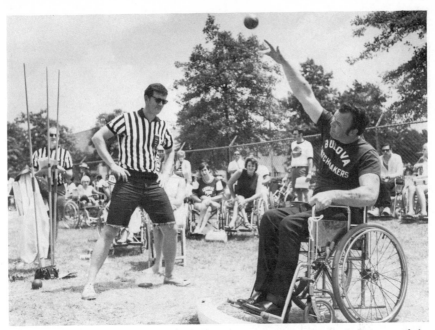

Track and field events can bring challenge to many of the handicapped. Courtesy of the AAHPER.

than 32 feet; the discus throw from a wheelchair was more than 126 feet. Most of these astonishing records have been broken since then.[5]

Other competitive events include slalom racing, archery (the FITA round, Columbia round, and the novice St. Nicholas round), dart archery (a combination of darts and archery), fencing (sabre, épée, foil), lawn bowling, pentathlon (javelin, shotput), snooker, swimming (front style,

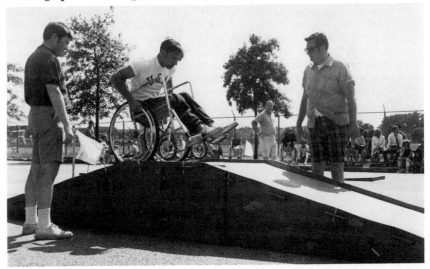

Slalom racing can also be done in wheelchairs. Courtesy of the AAHPER.

---

[5] Write to the N.C.A.A. for the most recent records.

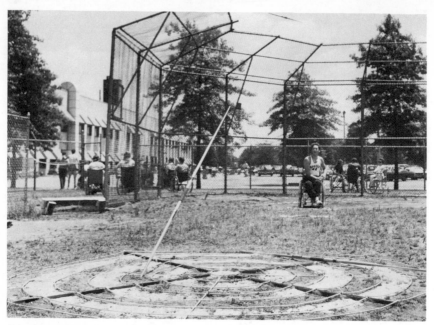

Practice makes perfect in learning any physical activity, but *only* if one practices perfectly. Courtesy of the National Wheelchair Athletic Association.

back freestyle, breaststroke, team relays), table tennis singles and doubles, and weight lifting.

Square dancing is enjoyed by thousands of wheelchair-bound persons. Because a wheelchair cannot be moved sideways, these movements are replaced by forward and back motions, and the square dance movement area is enlarged to ten or more feet in diameter.

> Right and left swings are done by having dancers hold onto their partner's right or left armrest. Momentum of the two individuals combines to produce a rotational motion which can be terminated simply by letting go. Honoring partners involves bringing chairs to face each other. Promenading is done with both members of each couple facing counterclockwise; gentlemen are nearer the center. Each dancer holds his partner's armrest while the lady provides most of the driving force with her right hand. In the circle four, each of the four gentlemen faces clockwise (for the right hand) and holds the nearer hand grip of the gentleman in front of him who is oriented ninety degrees relative to himself. The do-si-do is exactly the same as in any square dance except dancers turn chairs and move forward and backward until the move is completed.[6]

The Recreation Program

Increasingly, recreation programs for the orthopedically disabled are found in public-supported community centers. Many provide the use of their facilities for recreational purposes and leadership personnel as well as conducting the programs.

---

[6] "Wheelchair Square Dancing," *Journal of Health, Physical Education and Recreation* (November–December 1970), p. 96.

In addition, many voluntary agencies are expanding their programs to include the physically disabled. The national organization of Easter Seal Society, through its local chapters, have outstanding programs, and in some cities also sponsor activities for the homebound physically disabled. Service organizations such as the Chamber of Commerce, the Lion's Club, and the Rotary Club are likewise expanding their service programs to the crippled of all ages. Many conduct fund-raising events and publicize their activities through both radio and television.

Now we will discuss some of the major orthopedic disabilities separately.

AMPUTATIONS

One out of every 400 Americans has a major amputation of either arms or legs.[7] Amputations are classified as *congenital* (due to improper development), *traumatic* (due to accidents), or *elective* (in which the upper or lower extremities are removed by surgery because of a congenital or traumatic condition).

Most amputees wear a prosthetic appliance. An ingenious cosmetic prosthetic hand is often attached to an artificial arm; the hand is made movable by split hooks, steel cables, and a shoulder harness. An artificial foot and leg can be attached to a remaining stump for both appearance and utility. Children with amputations should be fitted for appliances as soon as possible in order to develop proper body alignment, and to

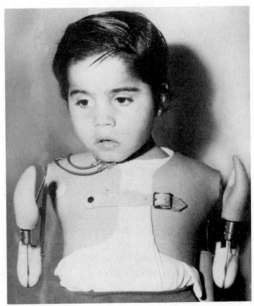

This child is fitted with artificial arms and hands. Courtesy of Rehabilitation International.

---

7 Howard Rusk, *Rehabilitation Medicine* (St. Louis: C. V. Mosby, 1964), p. 3.

learn how to move through space and support their own body weight, develop hand and foot dexterity, and develop proper hand-eye and foot-eye body coordination.

Adjustment Problems. Many amputees have phantom pains in the missing appendage that are very real and often cause both physiological and psychological difficulties. Comforting counseling is needed before, during, and after amputation procedures, for this is a truly traumatic experience. Top physical fitness should be maintained during each of these three periods. Isotonic bed exercises to build muscle tone and strength in the affected area should begin as soon as possible following surgery.

Implications for Physical Education. The physical rehabilitation program should be individualized and include (1) building and maintaining total fitness, (2) increasing the range of joint movements and body flexibility, (3) developing proficient appliance use, and (4) improving posture and body alignment for sitting and moving through space. Those using artificial legs must learn how to walk again; for those with artificial hands, training is necessary for proper manipulative development.

SPINAL BIFIDA

Spinal bifida is a birth defect that occurs in one out of every thousand births, with only 20 percent of the victims surviving the first year of life. In this congenital defect, the spinal column is not enclosed in the lower body, owing to a posterior fusion defect of the vertebral arches; this results in a malformation of the spinal column. This spinal separation is further complicated by tumor-like sacs on the spine. Anencephalus (a fetal monster having no brain) and this deformity are among the most common defects found in newborn infants.[8]

Adjustment Problems. Those afflicted may be paraplegics who must use wheelchairs, braces, or crutches. There are many degrees of involvement. Some victims can move about with relative ease, while others are far less mobile and more dependent upon others. They rarely have control of body elimination and must wear protective clothing and devices at all times. Because of their immobility, many develop serious postural and feet deformities and are often far behind their normal peers physically, socially, and academically.

Implications for Physical Education. The physical education program for persons with spinal bifida should be individually planned. Specific exercises to strengthen the upper part of the body should be given as prescribed by a physician. All kinds of social recreation activities such as cards, puzzles, tricks, and party games are especially suitable.

---

[8] James Wolf and Robert Anderson, *The Multiply Handicapped Child* (Springfield, Ill.: Charles Thomas, 1969), p. 67.

Because those afflicted have more leisure time than normal children (who take part in after-school lessons or activities), hobbies that can become progressively more challenging (such as photography or playing a musical instrument) are recommended.

ARTHRITIS

It is not uncommon to find that children, teenagers as well as adults, suffer from this malady; it is by no means confined to older people, although it is more prevalent among them.

Arthritis means inflammation of the joints. There are many kinds of arthritis, but 90 percent of those afflicted have one of the four main types: fibrositis, gout, osteo-arthritis, and rheumatoid arthritis.

Fibrositis is a term used for pain in muscle tendon and tissue around the joint. It does not involve real joint damage and is usually caused by exposure, injury, strain, or minor infection.

Gout pains result from strains, injuries, and/or excessive uric acid in the blood, causing swelling around a joint and making movement painful. Advanced cases can be crippling.

Osteo-arthritis is a gradual wearing-away of areas separating bone connections and even of the bones themselves. It usually is not as serious as other types of rheumatism, nor is it rapidly crippling. The weight-bearing joints such as the hips, spine, and knees are most usually affected. Enlarged end joints of fingers are common. Osteo-arthritis may develop as a result of joint trauma, inheritance, or advancing age. Usually it is very painful; the degree of pain varies, and the pain comes and goes in its earliest stage. Diet, weight reduction, heat and massage, and corrective muscle-training exercises to strengthen joint supports are frequently successful treatment measures.

Rheumatoid arthritis is the greatest crippler of all. It usually affects older people, but children often have it too. Luckily, today most of the crippling deformities of this disease can be prevented and, in some cases, arrested or controlled. In a high percentage of cases there is a temporary cure or arrest of its spread. Gold treatments, cortisone or similar steroids, ACTH, and blood transfusions are kinds of treatments most used.

Implications for Physical Education. Because excessive weight causes chronic joint stress and strain, the physical educator can do much to help persons afflicted with arthritis through an exercise and diet control program. Daily exercise programs given under the direction of a physician and the specialized physical educator will help in weight control and prevent faulty posture and flabby muscles. Both isometric and isotonic exercises can be used successfully, as can swimming in warm water, golf, badminton, archery, and tennis. Victims of this disease should also take part in recreational programs that will help rid them of their tensions, anxieties, and emotional strains. Yoga exercises are especially recommended, for they are both refreshing and relaxing.

MUSCULAR DYSTROPHY

This strange disease involves a chronic and progressive degeneration of the muscular system. In young children, it usually results in death before adulthood. It often begins in the muscles of the calves of the legs and then spreads symmetrically throughout the body. Most cases are inherited; only a few have unknown causes. This is a sex-linked disease that is only transmitted by the female. However, both females and males have the disease. Death usually results from suffocation due to malfunction of the muscles that control breathing. Although the actual number of persons afflicted by muscular dystrophy is unknown, it is estimated that 200,000 persons in the United States have it and that more than half of the cases are found in children ages 3 to 13 years.[9]

The most prevalent of the four types of this disease is *pseudohypertrophic dystrophy,* which is found in males three times as often as in females and between the ages of 3 and 10 years. It is inherited and is characterized by calf and forearm muscles that look greatly overdeveloped, though in actual fact, wasted muscle tissue has been replaced by fibrous tissue and fatty deposits. Victims have exceedingly poor coordination and have great difficulty in moving through space, sitting erect, and getting up from a sitting to a standing position. They also have a deformity due to atrophy of the spine, pelvic, and shoulder girdle areas of the body.

Juvenile muscular dystrophy affects both sexes equally and may appear any time in life. In this type there are general muscular weaknesses, which first appear just in the shoulder girdle area and then spreads throughout the whole body. However, most of those afflicted do reach middle age.

Facioscapulohumeral muscular dystrophy develops between the ages of 3 and 20 years. It appears first in the shoulders and upper arms, then spreads to the facial muscles. Victims typically have masklike faces and have difficulty in closing their eyes and in eating. The disease continues to spread throughout the body, affecting posture and body alignment. Although it is incurable, it spreads slowly, and many of its victims do reach maturity.

The fourth classification of this disease is made up of a mixture of several kinds, all of which are most likely to appear between the ages of 30 to 50 years, showing first in scapula and pelvic areas. Victims are irritable and tire easily as they become progressively weaker. They also lose hand-eye coordination, and because they have difficulty moving through space, remain shut-in isolates.

Adjustment Problems. Many children having muscular dystrophy are too sheltered by their parents and are behind their normal peers both physically and socially. All, however, have the same needs for security and belonging as do normal children. Some adults suffering from this malady tend to be shy and insecure; others are more outgoing. The atti-

---

[9] Daniel Arnheim, David Auster, and Walter Crowe, *Principles and Methods of Adapted Physical Education* (St. Louis: C. V. Mosby, 1969), p. 251.

tudes of family and friends toward them accounts for this difference in life outlook.

Implications for Physical Education. Because those with muscular dystrophy tend to be sedentary and overweight, physical activities are important and necessary. However, the kinds and amount of physical activities best suited to each individual should be based upon which of the four types of the disease he has, and all activities should be prescribed by a physician. Much can be done to prevent a certain amount of muscle deterioration and postural or other deformities through simple games and sports.

Light equipment is recommended, such as balloons instead of volleyballs, yarn or soft rubber instead of regulation softballs. Because many use crutches or are confined to wheelchairs, all activities included in the program will need much modification and should be conducted over several brief time periods rather than in one long one.

MUSCULOSKELETAL DIFFICULTIES

Many persons are injured while playing competitive games. Studies show that sprains rank first among those injuries, strains second. Most such injuries occur in the lower extremities of the body. Accidents in the home, going to and from school and at school, as well as those which occur at play, are the chief causes of death among children. They are also a serious threat to teenagers and young adults. Often it is the school nurse or athletic trainer who is called in to give first aid to the injured, but most frequently it is the school physical educator or recreation leader. Consequently, training of such people should include courses in first aid, athletic injury, and adaptive physical education and recreation for the handicapped. Injured students are frequently placed in an adaptive physical education course for a whole semester or temporarily. Providing activities that are best suited to speed recovery is the physical educator's task. Recreational opportunities for the handicapped are increasing rapidly at the present time throughout the nation.

Many students have chronic or congenital musculoskeletal disorders. In 1960 there were 1,950,000 orthopedically handicapped persons below the age of 21, and a predicted 2,425,000 in 1970.[10] Some of these persons have congenital birth defects, others have temporary or chronic conditions.

The next section of this chapter is concerned with posture deviations, which can result in musculoskeletal difficulties.

POSTURE DEVIATIONS

The most common posture deviations and faulty body mechanics are: (1) *kyphosis* (round shoulders), (2) *lordosis* (hollow back with a

---

10 *Health of Children of School Age,* U.S. Department of Health, Education and Welfare, Children's Bureau, Washington, D.C., 1964, p. 18.

protruding rear), (3) *scoliosis* (crooked back or S-curve of the vertebral column), (4) *forward head tilt,* (5) *protruding shoulder blades,* (6) *faulty foot mechanics,* and (7) *flat feet.* All of these difficulties can be classified either as *structural* (permanent) deviations or *functional disorders* (correctable). Functional disorders are caused by improper functioning of the muscles and ligaments of the body. Every person has individual rhythmic movement patterns and limitations, body build, and personality traits; and how a person moves is most significant to a well-trained observer. Plato said that the most beautiful motion is the one that achieves the best results with the least effort; and because the body houses the soul, it should be kept beautiful. Actually, there are many postures the body assumes in sitting, walking, and moving through space, or standing still—not just the one static body position most laymen call "posture."

For beauty of movement, the body should be balanced over its foundation base (the feet) and center of gravity (slightly above the hips). Like a set of well-laid blocks placed into a balanced slightly curved position, each body part should be perfectly balanced over the feet, hips, and chest. A quick test for good posture can be made by dropping a weighted line from the tip of a person's right ear down below the right knee. If the posture is good, the line will bisect the shoulder, hip, side of the leg at the knee joint, and ankle. The head should be perfectly balanced over the neck, and shoulders should be relaxed and held down, each pointing directly to the side. The chest should be held high and relaxed, stomach and rear pulled in, the knees held loose and relaxed.

Walking, which is one of our best means of daily cost-free exercise, requires a constant shifting of balance; walking is an alternate loss and recovery of balance. As one leg swings forward with the heel striking first, the rear foot and leg push forward and body weight transfers to the forward foot in a continuously interchanging movement. The most common walking defects are exhibited in Figure 6–1: (a) the "spraddle-footed, toes-out waddler"; (b) the pidgeon-toed; (c) the "arm-thrasher," who pumps along through space; (d) the "bounding head-bobber"; (e) the

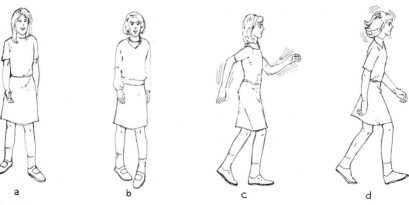

a   b   c   d

Fig. 6–1

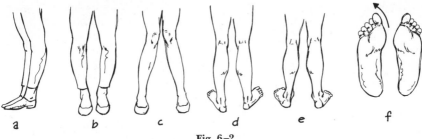

Fig. 6–2

"heel thrower-outer"; (f) the "lost coin-searcher," whose head stays down; (g) the "stomper"; (h) the "shuffler"; and (i) the "bent-kneed high-heel bobber," whose Achilles tendon has become shortened from wearing high heels for too long a period and who walks with legs flexed.

Hammer toes, corns, bunions, and flat or high arches cause aching feet and faulty movement problems. The most common leg and foot faults are shown in Figure 6–2: (a) back-knees, (b) bow-legs, (c) knock-knees, (d) ankle pronatation, (e) ankle suppination and bulging ankle bones, (f) big toe turned out.

Adjustment Problems. Those with posture problems sometimes also have adjustment problems. Many feel inferior and self-conscious. Some try to compensate for these feelings by becoming loud-mouthed, hostile, and aggressive; others become withdrawn and shy. Poor posture can be either the *cause* of such adjustment problems or the result. In any event, correction can help an individual look better and develop a more positive self-image. Frequently counseling is also needed for emotional problems.

Implications for Physical Education. This program should consist of sports and games plus corrective exercises. The former should entail both individual and pair activities as well as team games. Because many victims of poor posture are uncoordinated, efforts should be made to teach them

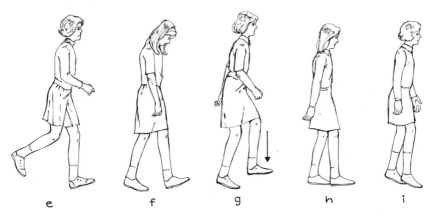

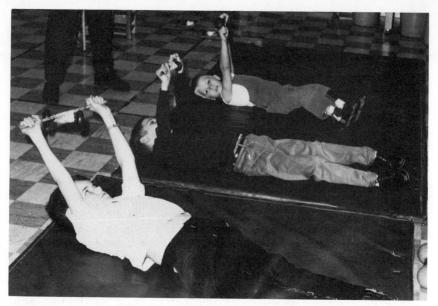

Children with posture problems can develop hand, arm, and shoulder girdle strength through special exercise programs. Courtesy of the AAHPER.

skills and guide them toward activities through which they can learn better posture and control.

Corrective exercises should be given under the direction of a physician or physical education specialist. Because pure exercise programs can soon become dull, adding music and conducting the class on a small individualized group basis will add interest. Following are some activities and exercises that can be used in physical education and recreational programs for those with poor posture.[11]

For a Forward Head

1. Lie prone on the floor. Press back of neck firmly down and feel the motion. Relax and repeat 10 to 20 times.
2. Lie supine on the floor with arms outstretched. On 1, lift head up high. On 2 and 3 turn it to the right and left. Down on 4. Repeat.
3. Circle head first to right, then left; then left to right. Next tuck chin as far as it will go, then tilt head back as much as possible. Repeat. Add resistance by placing one hand on head, trying to prevent movement.
4. Hold a towel taut behind head and push neck hard against it. Relax and repeat 10 times.
5. Sit up very straight. Take a deep breath, cross arms and grasp each arm firmly as you push against the wall. Relax and repeat.

For Round Shoulders, Round Back, and Protruding Shoulder Blades

1. Stand tall. On 1 swing arms across body. On 2 stretch them as high as possible and stand on tiptoes. On 3 return to place. Repeat 10 times.

---

[11] All of these exercises should be tried out first by the reader, so that instructing others in such activities will be based on first-hand knowledge of the teacher.

2. Sit with crossed legs with hands clasped in back of neck. On 1 bend trunk forward. On 2 slowly straighten spine, giving resistance with hands clasped at neck. On 3 sit up tall and extend back. Repeat 10 times.

3. Sit with legs crossed, arms held straight out to sides, and head up. On 1 make small circles, with arms going clockwise on 2. On 3 make big circle going clockwise and counterclockwise on count 4. Repeat 10 times.

4. Stand with flexed elbows out to the sides and with fingers interlocked in front of body. On 1 try to pull right hand away from left, which tries to prevent this. Relax on 2. Repeat.

For the Correction of Round Shoulders (lordosis)

1. Lying on back, clasp flexed legs. On 1 pull legs as close to chest as possible. On 2 extend both legs together up as high as possible. On 3 return them to chest. On 4 lower them. Repeat movements.

2. Lie in a prone position with hands behind head. On 1 raise head and elbows. On 2 return to place. Repeat.

3. Sit with crossed legs and arms to sides. On 1 take a deep breath and round the shoulders as much as possible. On 2 exhale and move arms and shoulders back as far as possible. Repeat.

4. Sit with legs flexed and hands clasped behind neck. On 1 twist body and touch right elbow to left knee and try to push upper body and neck back as far as possible while clasped hands push forward to prevent the movement. On 3 twist to touch left elbow to right knee. On 4 return to place.

5. Sit cross-legged and erect with arms above head. Arms, head, and back are against the wall. On 1, 2, 3, and 4, gradually lower arms down the wall until hands are opposite head. Keep back pressed to the wall. Raise arms back to position on counts 5, 6, 7, and 8.

For the Correction of Scoliosis (the S curve of the vertebral column)

1. Kneel on right knee with left leg out to the side and right arm over head. On 1 bend trunk to the right and stretch it as far as possible. On 2 return to place. Switch positions and on 3 bend left. On 4 return to place. (This should only be done on the right side for a marked left curve or vice versa. It may be done on both sides, if the abnormality is only slight.)

2. Stand with right foot on a stool or chair with left arm pointing to the right over head. On 1 bring trunk to the right and twist it back as far as possible to bring head forward to touch right knee. Return to place on 2. Repeat on the other side.

3. Get into a crawling position on a mat or rug. Creep forward, stretching the right arm and left knee forward on 1. Stretch left arm and right knee forward on 2. Repeat, going forward, then going in circles.

4. Lie in a supine position with knees flexed and a helper holding feet, or put them under a heavy chair. Stretch body as much as possible with arms overhead and toes stretched forward on count 1. On 2 come to a sitting position. On 3 return to place and relax. Repeat.

5. Hang with body in full extension from a bar or rings and hold this position as long as possible.

PROBLEMS OF THE FEET AND ANKLES

The foot is an example of masterful engineering, for although it is composed of only twenty-six small bones, it is so constructed that the total weight of the body can be well supported on three small areas—the base of the big and little toes and the heel. There are seven ankle bones, the largest and strongest of which is that of the heel; all these tiny foot bones are held in place by strong ligaments, muscles, and tendons over the longitudinal and transverse arches.

A variety of afflictions affect the feet. When body weight is incorrectly balanced, the result is ankle supination (weight carried on the outer foot borders) or ankle pronation (weight carried on the inner foot borders). Because the feet are farthest from the heart, circulatory problems often show up first in swollen feet and ankles. Shoes, especially those with high heels, are hard on the arches, for the extra elevation of the heel relieves the calf muscles of their function of supporting the longitudinal arch, causing it gradually to weaken. They also cause a redistribution of body weight, pushing it forward on the arch and spreading the toes. Consequently, those who wear high heels should do foot exercises often and change to low heels or walk around barefooted for a while every day. For serious foot difficulties, one should seek the services of a medical orthopedic specialist or podiatrist. Corns, bunions, hammertoes, and ingrown toenails result from wearing improperly fitting shoes; trench foot and athlete's foot are signs of faulty foot hygiene.

Implications for Physical Education. The physical educator should be able to recognize foot problems in students. Those whose feet and legs tire easily will be unable to do well in the program unless they are helped to remedy the causes. Following are some helpful exercises for strengthening feet and ankles.

EXERCISES

The Alphabet Writer

Sit in a chair with legs crossed. Swing free foot to write the letters A to M (Figure 6–3). Cross legs the other way and finish writing the rest of the alphabet with the other foot.

Tiptoe Position

Standing straight with arms extended at sides, focus eyes on a spot across the room. Raise body slowly to tiptoe position, then slowly lower body. Do 10 times.

The Heel Lifter

Curl toes over a large book such as a telephone directory, standing tall. Raise and lower body slowly (Figure 6–4). Do 10 times.

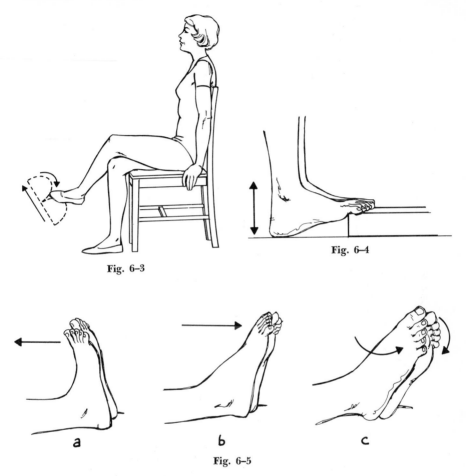

Fig. 6–3

Fig. 6–4

Fig. 6–5

Back and Out Foot Exercise

Sit barefooted on floor with legs together and extended, feet in relaxed position. Bring both feet back toward you (Figure 6–5a), then return to relaxed position (Figure 6–5b). Turn soles toward each other (Figure 6–5c) without using your hands for assistance, and pat them 10 times. Repeat whole pattern, first slowly, then as fast as possible, 10 times.

The Toe Curl

Sit barefooted on floor with legs extended and feet together. On 1, spread toes far apart as possible. Relax on 2. On 3, curl toes under (Figure 6–6); relax on 4. Do 10 times.

The Pencil Pickup

Seated in a chair, pick up a pencil with bare toes. Write your full name on a piece of paper and repeat with other foot (Figure 6–7). Or, using toes, pick up 10 marbles, one at a time, and put them in a box.

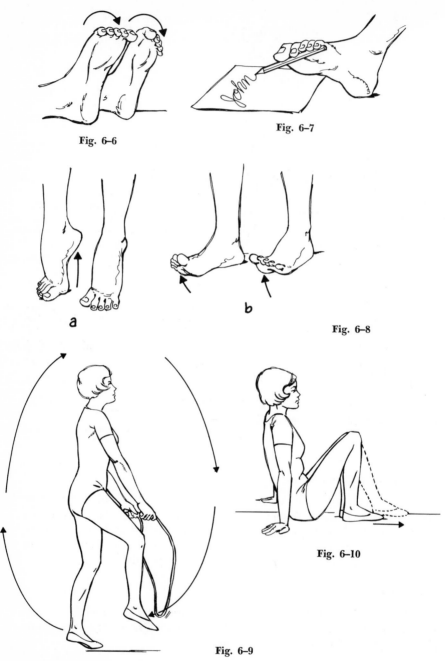

Fig. 6–6

Fig. 6–7

a

b

Fig. 6–8

Fig. 6–10

Fig. 6–9

Toes Up and Down

Stand erect with bare feet apart. On 1, rise on toes (Figure 6–8a); 2, lower body. On 3, lift front part of each foot (Figure 6–8b); lower on 4. Do 15 times.

Rope Jumping

Skip rope in place 25 times, clearing rope with one foot at a time, first springing from toes, then transferring weight to back of foot (Figure 6–9). Next jump with feet together, springing from toes. Work up to doing this 50, 75, and finally 100 times.

The Up and Back Toe Crawl

Sit with heels drawn up close to the hips, bare feet and knees together, palms on the floor. Keeping feet on floor, advance feet by toe movement for 10 counts, then back (Figure 6–10). Do 20 times.

SUGGESTED READINGS

ADAMS, RONALD, *Games, Sports and Exercises for the Physically Handicapped.* Philadelphia: Lea & Febiger, 1972.

Boy Scouts of America, *Scouting for the Physically Handicapped.* North Brunswick, N.J., 08902.

CRATTY, BRYANT, *Active Learning: Games to Enhance Academic Abilities.* Englewood Cliffs, N.J.: Prentice-Hall, 1971.

KRAUS, HANS, and WELHELEN ROAB, *Hypokinetic Disease.* Springfield, Ill.: Charles Thomas, 1961.

LOWMAN, CHARLES, and CARL YOUNG, *Postural Fitness.* Philadelphia: Lea & Febiger, 1960.

PETTIL, MILTON, "Physical Education for Orthopedically Handicapped Children," *Journal of Health, Physical Education and Recreation* (February 1971), p. 75.

SAGE, GEORGE, *Introduction to Motor-Behavior: A Neuropsychological Approach.* Reading, Mass.: Addison-Wesley, 1971.

STEIN, THOMAS, and DOUGLAS SESSOMS, *Recreation and Special Population.* Boston: Holbrook Press, 1973.

VODOLA, THOMAS, *Individualized Physical Education Programs.* Englewood Cliffs, N.J.: Prentice-Hall, 1973.

Suggested Films

Two 16MM, sound-color, documentary films—"Paralympics London" (15 minutes) and "Paralympics Israel 1968" (12 minutes)—show competition by men and women with paraplegia and post-polio paraplegia in such events as swimming, track and field, weight lifting, fencing, archery, darchery (a form of precision archery), lawn bowling, ping pong, slalom, pentathlon, and wheelchair basketball. The films show the adapted sports program, both nationally and internationally, while conveying the story of rehabilitation. Information about purchase and rental of these films can be obtained from the Chairman, United States Wheelchair Sports Fund, 40-24 62nd Street, Woodside, N.Y. 11377.

Wheelchair Sports Information

Periodicals and Publications

Accent on Living (quarterly), 802 Reinthaler, Bloomington, Ill. 61701.

Caliper (monthly), 153 Lyndhurst Avenue, Toronto, Ontario, Canada.

NAPH National Newsletter (quarterly), National Association of the Physically Handicapped, 2 Meetinghouse Road, Reedsferry, N.H. 03078.

National Wheelchair Athletic Association Newsletter, 40-24 62nd Street, Woodside, N.Y. 11377.

Paraplegic News (monthly), 935 Coastline Drive, Seal Beach, Cal. 90740.

Sigma Signs, Delta Sigma Omicron (Alpha Chapter), Room 130, Rehabilitation-Education Center, Oak Street and Stadium Drive, Champaign, Ill. 61820.

A Special Report on Organizing Wheelchair Sporting Events in Your City, 1466 Lafayette Street, Lincoln Park, Mich. 48146.

Games

Alabama Wheelchair Games, 709 Pleasant Grove Road, Pleasant Grove, Ala. 35127.

Arizona Wheelchair Games, 4501 West Indian School Road, Phoenix, Ariz. 85031.

Bay State Wheelchair Games, 6 Elizabeth Lane, Peabody, Mass. 01960.

California Wheelchair Games, 500 Hendon Court, Sunnyvale, Cal. 94087.

Davenport-Iowa Wheelchair Games, 1776 44th Street, Rock Island, Ill. 61201.

Lakewood Wheelchair Games, 5939 E. South Street, Apartment 4, Lakewood, Cal. 90713.

Michigan Wheelchair Games, 1466 Lafayette Street, Lincoln Park, Mich. 48146.

National Wheelchair Games, 40-24 62nd Street, Woodside, N.Y. 11377.

New England Wheelchair Games, Crotched Mountain Rehabilitation Center, Greenfield, N.H. 03078.

Pennsylvania Wheelchair Games, Highland Elementary School, 1325 Carlisle Road, Camp Hill, Pa. 17011.

Stoke-Mandeville Paralympic Games, Stoke-Mandeville Spinal Cord Injuries Center, Aylesbury, England.

Organizations (Contact national associations for information about state and/or local affiliates.)

American Wheelchair Bowling Association, Route #2, Box 750, Lutz, Fla. 33549.

Indoor Sports Club, 3445 Trumbull Street, San Diego, Cal. 92106.

National Association of the Physically Handicapped, 1466 Lafayette Street, Lincoln Park, Mich. 48146.

National Paraplegia Foundation, 333 North Michigan Avenue, Chicago, Ill. 60601.

National Wheelchair Athletic Association, 40-24 62nd Street, Woodside, N.Y. 11377.

National Wheelchair Basketball Association, Rehabilitation-Education Center, Oak Street and Stadium Drive, University of Illinois, Champaign, Ill. 61820.

Paralyzed Veterans of America, 3636 16th Street, N.W., Washington, D.C. 20010 (national office: Peter L. Lassen, executive director). Sports coordinator: John W. Ebert, 956 Henhawk Road, Baldwin, N.Y. 11510.

Individual Contacts

Benjamin H. Lipton, founder and chairman, National Wheelchair Athletic Association, 40-24 62nd Street, Woodside, N.Y. 11377.

Mariann Soulek, special services supervisor, King County Park Department, 430 S. 156th Street, Seattle, Wash. 98148.

Timothy J. Nugent, director, Division of Rehabilitation-Education Services, University of Illinois, Oak Street and Stadium Drive, Champaign, Ill. 61820.

Stefan Florescu, 1466 Lafayette Street, Lincoln Park, Mich. 48146.

Richard Switzer, principal, Human Resources Center, Albertson, N. Y. 11507.

Julian U. Stein, consultant, Programs for the Handicapped, AAHPER, 1201 16th Street, N.W., Washington, D.C. 20036.

7

Mental Illness

In most hospitals and clinics mentally ill and emotionally disturbed patients are served by a group of experts from several professions. This team is usually made up of a psychiatrist; a psychiatric social or case worker; a clinical psychologist; nurses; a psychometrist who gives, scores, and records a number of psychological tests; and one or more recreational and occupational therapists.

In this chapter, the discussion will be on those people who suffer in varying degrees from emotional and mental disturbances. A sharp line will not be drawn between serious mental illness and the psychoneuroses; it is acknowledged that those who suffer from all degrees of such malfunctioning can be aided by specific programs of physical education and recreational therapy. Nor will we here deal with that large category made up of people born with mental limitations (even though specific programs are beneficial to them as well). Instead, the types of programs needed will be stressed, the training necessary to adequately provide them, and the reasons behind the importance of physical and recreational activity for those who are the victims of emotional handicaps—from the mildly neurotic individual to the hospitalized psychotic.

The reader may also notice the preponderance of the term "recreation" in this chapter. It is assumed here that you will know that this also refers to physical education activities; but in discussing mental illness, physical education is practised primarily with a recreational overtone.

Characteristics

Our own era in the history of mankind is often referred to as "The Age of Anxiety" or "The Century of Waste." It is no wonder, then, that mental illness and emotional disturbances are increasing at such an alarming rate in our nation. It is estimated by authorities in this field that one out of every five or six people in the United States suffers from some serious type of behavior disorder. It is also claimed that 52 percent of all persons hospitalized are for mental illness, and that one out of every ten Americans will become seriously mentally ill at some time during his life. It is also estimated that between 10 and 14 percent of elementary school children are emotionally disturbed, and about 400 out of 100,000 children under 18 require psychiatric care as out-patients each year.[1]

CLASSIFICATION

The mentally ill can be roughly fit into the following categories:

Functional psychoses. This group involves around 1 million cases; it includes schizophrenia, manic-depressive psychosis, involutional reactions, and paranoid conditions.

Organic conditions. In this group are another 1 million patients who suffer from acute and chronic brain disturbances accompanied by abnormal behavior.

Mental deficiency. There are 4 million in this category who are feeble-minded.

Conduct disorders. This group is made up of 5 million or more disturbed persons who "act out" their adjustment and personality problems. It includes drug addicts, alcoholics, sexual deviates, sociopaths, and psychopaths.[2]

Psychoneuroses. It is estimated that 8 to 10 million children and adults have psychoneurotic disorders. These include phobias, compulsions, conversion, hysteria, etc.

Psychosomatic disorders. This is the largest group and is conservatively estimated to be around 20 million. Included in it are those who suffer from high blood pressure, ulcers, asthma, and allergic conditions. These individuals are not mentally ill or greatly emotionally disturbed, but do have physical conditions caused by worry, tension, the environment in which they live, or a combination of any of these factors.

There are numerous reasons why mental illness is on the increase in our nation. Some authorities believe that this problem is indirectly caused by "bigness," or the crowding of more and more people into fewer and fewer places to the degree that a person loses his concept of

---

1 Carl Willgoose, *Health Education in the Elementary School* (Philadelphia: W. B. Saunders, 1974), p. 9.

2 Alcoholism is increasing rapidly in our country and now makes up our most pressing health and social-civic problem among adults, college students, and younger teenagers. It is rapidly becoming a problem among children in the sixth, seventh, and eighth grades.

himself as a unique human being. Others believe that the problem is indirectly caused by boredom, sameness, and ugliness; that we may be losing contact with the beauty of nature and the land as we increasingly cover our green fields and open spaces with cement, destroy and pollute our environment by industrial and personal waste products. Ecologists now claim that unless this mutilation of the environment is halted, man cannot survive on this earth for more than a few centuries.

Medical authorities classify the mentally ill into two major divisions: those with disorders of the brain, such as brain damage, and those with disorders of a psychogenic origin—these latter have no apparent physical causes (e.g., acute anxiety, alcoholism, advanced drug addiction or marked antisocial destructive behavior). Recent scientific research has disclosed that some kinds of insanity are brought about by biochemical and electrochemical imbalance.

The mentally ill may or may not seek help for their illness. Some are ill enough to be hospitalized; of these, many are no danger to others while some are a danger to themselves and to others and thus must be segregated from society. These are people whose illness prevents them from distinguishing between right and wrong, and whose actions are irrational and destructive. Milder emotional disturbances can often be treated by psychiatry or psychotherapy while the patient carries on a fairly normal life.

Some definition of terms related to mental illness will be helpful at this point.

Adjunctive therapists—recreation leaders, occupational therapists, or other members of a rehabilitation team.

Insanity—a legal term meaning that a person does not know right from wrong and needs to be in legal custody or guardianship for his own protection and that of society.

Manic-depressive psychosis—a major behavior disorder characterized by varying moods from mental elation to mental depression.

Paranoia—a disorder characterized by delusions and strange fears that one's life is in danger.

Psychiatric social or case worker—one who works with and collects pertinent information about a mental patient and is a liaison between him and his family and friends.

Psychology—the science of behavior focusing upon human beings and their behavior and relationships with others.

Psychosis—a major mental illness in which a person loses touch with reality. This may be due to a functional or learned response or be organic resulting from a brain injury. The victim is often dangerous to himself and society.

Psychotherapy—counseling and other techniques used by a psychiatrist or clinical psychologist in the treatment of behavior disorders.

Schizophrenia—one of the functional psychoses characterized by apathy and withdrawal from reality.

Teaching Suggestions

It is imperative that the physical and recreational therapist know the type and source of behavior disorder of each person in his group. Activities should be selected for each member from a written prescription by a psychiatrist. For example, such a prescription might be to provide activities in which the docile person would have to engage in games in which he must show aggression (as in power volleyball) or would have to learn to work well with others (as in singing in a choir or playing bridge with a partner).

It is important for the recreational and physical education therapist to realize that in most instances of mental illness, the earliest and most significant symptoms are seen in a disturbance in play and recreation patterns. These include the inability to sleep and/or relax, fear of being with and competing against others, and a compulsive need to "keep busy and work hard." And the first signs of recovery from mental illness is seen when patients begin to want to play and be with other people again.

Dr. Alexander Reid Martin, an eminent psychiatrist, has said:

> Recreation plays a significant role in preserving health and maintaining the status quo, in preventing and treating disease and in bringing man back to himself. Recreation in its truest sense should serve to bring healthy man forward to a new self.[3]

Through play the abnormal as well as the normal can find their needs for love and security fulfilled. Through play they can also learn how to replace reality escape mechanisms such as regression, introversion, segregation, rationalization, dissociation, or projection with a more positive type of behavior through which is gained greater self-control, self-realization, and personal insight.

Another valuable knowledge for those concerned with physical therapy and recreation for the mentally ill is that *every person needs recognition*. Some gain this in socially approved ways, others through negative behavior, for it is better to be recognized as being "bad" than not to be noticed at all. All persons, regardless of age, should receive praise for trying to improve, whether this be to improve behavior or gain skill mastery.

It is common for emotionally disturbed people to "give up"—not respond to challenges. In more extreme cases of mental disturbance, individuals sometimes suddenly go into destructive rages and must be physically or chemically restrained. A skilled recreation therapist can aid in enticing both types of people slowly into substituting positive for negative behavior through physical activities. This can be accomplished by encouraging each patient to work out his feelings through

---

[3] "Professional Attitudes and Practices," *Recreation for the Mentally Ill*, a conference report (Washington, D.C.: AAHPER, 1958), p. 17.

such program offerings as art, music, or sports. When inactivity is replaced with activity, the depressed person often responds to the challenge of activities which other patients are enjoying. Games should be provided which will "allow" hostile, destructive patients to let off steam through noisy, big-muscle activities.

Every person needs to develop self-control and independence. Although many of the mentally ill regress to childish behavior, lack self-control, and have marked dependence upon the recreation therapist, each patient must learn to grow up emotionally. He must patiently be guided by words, physical contact, and through program activities to become more responsible for the consequences of his own actions. Each patient must feel that the recreation leader *wants* him to improve and is helping him to master self-control as well as new physical skills. He must also develop confidence in his ability to learn to do things for and by himself.

Training of Physical Education and Recreation Leaders

The field of therapeutic physical education and recreation for the mentally ill and emotionally disturbed has two levels: the administrative supervisory and the activity level. Professional preparation should include field work and internship in a hospital or clinic. The Veterans Administration's Student Affiliate Recreation Trainee Program is an example of such a professional program.

The undergraduate program should be broad and consist of two years of liberal arts which include the humanities; the social behavioral, physical, and biological sciences; and program skills. Special emphasis should be given to the field of psychology. Field work experiences should be provided in cooperation with many mental health agencies. The degree requirements should also include research projects in both psychology per se and the psychology of recreation.

On the graduate level the curriculum should focus on hospital recreation. It should include:

1. The understanding of illness and their psychological effects
2. Medical and psychiatric information
3. Skills in recreation planning based upon patients' needs and interests while in a hospital
4. Effective use of community resources
5. Knowledge and practice in the role of the recreation leader as a part of the hospital team and psychiatric staff
6. Development of proper attitudes
7. Interpretation of job responsibilities
8. Knowledge and practice in group processes and dynamics
9. Knowledge and application of behavioral sciences

10. Research and evaluation

11. Understanding of the psychological aspects of leisure [4]

The program should also include an internship in a hospital and the student should work only with a supervisor who has had hospital recreation experience.

An example of the many clinical training opportunities which are available for students interested in becoming specialists in hospital recreation is this one from the Timberlawn Psychiatric Center, a private hospital in Dallas, Texas, which has an outstanding therapeutic recreational program:

CLINICAL TRAINING PROGRAMS [5]

Clinical training programs are offered in all of the major professional disciplines represented on the hospital staff. As a part of overall hospital policy, it is believed that a teaching hospital is a better hospital. Expenditures for student stipends are justified on the premise that such educational programs ultimately improve the quality of patient care.

In the Department of Recreation Therapy, clinical affiliations are offered in Music Therapy and in Recreation Therapy.

MUSIC THERAPY

The clinical training course in Music Therapy is established at Timberlawn Psychiatric Hospital to enable the students to fulfill requirements for a degree in Music Therapy from approved universities and thereby qualify for registration in the National Association for Music Therapy. The program is organized on two levels.

Hospital Orientation (three months)

Students presently enrolled in Music Therapy at approved universities are eligible to serve an aideship of three months duration in the hospital. The goals of this activity are: the orientation of the student to the hospital atmosphere, the development of observation and leadership qualities through patient contact and through association with staff members, and the gleaning of techniques and information which will be applicable to the future studies of the music therapy student.

Clinical Affiliation (six months)

Timberlawn Psychiatric Hospital is also qualified to provide a psychiatric internship in Music Therapy which allows the candidate for a degree in Music Therapy an opportunity for six months of uninterrupted experience in the use of music in a psychiatric setting.

Objectives in this program include: individual and group treatment of patients assigned to various music therapy activities, the understanding of the administration and operation of departments in the psychiatric hospital, the orientation to medical and psychiatric concepts pertinent to the

---

[4] Ibid., pp. 22–23.

[5] For further information, write to the Director of Recreation Therapy, Timberlawn Psychiatric Hospital, P.O. Box 11288, Dallas, Texas 75223.

treatment of patients, the approximation of a normal job situation, the assignment of leadership responsibilities designed to help the student gain added maturity and new insights into his field and his place in it.

During this training period, the student is supervised by a Registered Music Therapist whose responsibility is to assess the progress of the student and become aware of his developing needs. A close association with the Music Therapy Department Head at the student's university is maintained by written reports sent periodically by the training supervisor. Personal visits by the university personnel are encouraged whenever possible.

Evaluations of the student's work are written by the Music Therapist and Recreation Therapy staff with enough frequency to provide a tangible scale of student progress. In order to provide increased communication skills, the student is also expected to prepare a variety of oral and written reports on activities observed and organized.

At the termination of the internship, final evaluations are written by the Timberlawn staff members and an evaluation is sent to the music professor at the student's university.

The student is given an affidavit to the effect that his clinical affiliation has been completed satisfactorily. This affidavit may be used for his application for registration as a Registered Music Therapist with the National Association for Music Therapy.

Currently, clinical affiliations in Music Therapy are established with the University of Kansas (Lawrence, Kansas), Michigan State University (East Lansing, Michigan), University of Wisconsin (Oshkosh, Wisconsin), Texas Woman's University (Denton, Texas), and Lincoln University (Jefferson City, Missouri).

THE PHYSICAL ACTIVITIES PROGRAM

Dr. Paul Haun, a nationally recognized psychiatrist interested in recreational therapy, has devised the following eight indices by which the effectiveness of recreation services to mentally ill patients can be measured:

1. Increased number of patients attending
2. Increased patient responsiveness as observers or participants
3. Increased identification with a group in team games
4. Higher level of sportsmanship in competitive games
5. Greater facility and improved quality of performance in individual recreational pursuits
6. Increased number of patients seeking instruction in performance skills
7. Movement of the static patient population from simpler to more complex recreative activities
8. More frequent expression and choice by the patients [6]

The best recreation programs (which of course includes physical education) for the mentally ill are diversified and meet the interests of the majority of patients but at the same time provide recreational outlets

---

[6] *Recreation, A Medical Viewpoint* (New York: Bureau of Publications, Teachers College, Columbia University, 1965), p. 70.

for smaller groups and more seriously ill individuals. These programs (1) are properly balanced between regularly scheduled activities and special events, (2) help participants gain increased skills in crafts and sports, (3) fully utilize community resources for outings or other purposes, and (4) provide outlets for feelings of aggression as well as creativity. Above all, the program should be under the direction of a specialist in therapeutic recreation.

Suggested program activities for this group are:

Active Games
  Volleyball
  Croquet
  Shuffleboard
  Bowling
  Badminton
  Tether ball
  Table shuffleboard
  Lawn bowling

Social Recreation
  Games parties
  Night clubs
  Monte Carlos
  Tournaments
  Quiz programs
  Picnics and barbecues
  Dances
  Masquerades
  Movies
  Family nights

Dramatic and Language Activities
  Skits
  Floor shows
  Puppets
  Story telling and story reading
  Panel discussions
  Publication of a hospital newspaper

Combative Activities
  Highly active and noisy games
  Punching Bag
  Boxing
  Wrestling

Off-Grounds Activities
  Excursions
  Golf
  Fishing
  Boating and water skiing
  Concerts
  Plays
  Sports events

Quiet Games
  Puzzles
  Bridge

  Forty-Two
  Checkers
  Cribbage
  Chess
  Poker
  Canasta
  Scrabble
  Chinese checkers
  Bingo
  Yacht

Dancing
  Folk and square dancing
  Ballroom dancing
  Creative dance

Aquatics
  Swimming
  Diving
  Lifesaving
  Boating (combined with fishing)

Special Holiday Celebrations
  Hallowe'en
  Thanksgiving
  Christmas
  New Year's
  July 4th

Music
  Group singing
  Rhythm bands
  Music listening
  Choral groups

Work Activities
  Care of facilities
  Care and repair of equipment
  Typing and mimeographing
  Cleaning office and recreational
    areas
  Shopping for supplies
  Meal planning
  Cooking
  Setting tables, serving, clean-up of
    food
  Preparing for cookouts and parties
  Sewing

Throughout the country there are many excellent programs of therapeutic recreation, which counteract hospital monotony; offer satisfying and enjoyable experiences; replace inactivity and aid in preventing physical deterioration; contribute to the patients' ultimate adjustment at home, in the community, and vocationally; and provide a variety of stimulating recreational activities in a group setting.

Although the field of therapeutic recreation is new, it is gaining in importance. It has a challenging future in our society, in which so many people are struggling with varying degrees of emotional disturbances and mental illnesses.

Emotionally Disturbed Children

Before ending this chapter, some mention should be made of the serious and special problem of emotional disturbances in the very young. It is estimated that 10 to 12 percent of all children have maladjustment and emotional problems requiring psychiatric help. Experts claim that in a class of 32 pupils, 3 to 4 will have emotional problems, and one will need psychiatric assistance.[7] The need is clear for more research that places emphasis on prevention. More money is also needed to train and hire qualified people to work with these children who often hate (fight reaction) or are withdrawn (the flight reaction). Recreation is now being used as an effective therapeutic tool for these individuals. Types of recreational services available to the emotionally disturbed are conducted on both an in- and out-patient basis.

Dr. Fritz Redl, one recognized expert in this field, suggests that recreation for disturbed children is primarily a drain for damaging impulses. It also serves as a frustration avoidance by giving the child the quick reward of fun and success, helps children through group pressure to try new and different activities and thus broaden their experiences, and provides each child with depersonalized controls. As Dr. Redl has discovered, such children can best learn through games that rules are a vital part of success in life as well as in play.

Guiding principles for planning programs for disturbed children are to

1. Help the children become contributing members of society
2. Give opportunities for immediate satisfaction and feelings of progress by tailoring the activities to the specific achievement levels of each group member
3. Make the activities a stimulant for further related activity
4. Gear the activities to the real interests of the group

The recreation specialist in this field must work closely with a psychiatrist, case worker, and other youth specialists. There must be full

---

[7] Harold Cornacchia, Wesley Staton, and Leslie Irwin, *Health in Elementary Schools*, 3rd ed. (St. Louis: C. V. Mosby, 1970), p. 316.

access to all records so that the specialist can learn as much as possible about each child. Then with great love and utmost patience, a recreation program can be provided that is planned and taught so that these unhappy youngsters may be best helped.

SUGGESTED READINGS

American Association for Health, Physical Education and Recreation, *Recreation for the Mentally Ill* (a conference report). Washington, D.C.: AAHPER, 1959.

AXLINE, VIRGINIA, *Play Therapy*, rev. ed. New York: Ballantine Books, 1969.

GELLHORN, E., and G. N. LOOFBURROW, *Emotions and Emotional Disorders*. New York: Harper & Row, 1963.

HAUN, PAUL, *Recreation; a Medical Viewpoint*. New York: Bureau of Publications, Columbia University, 1965.

KRAUS, HANS, *Therapeutic Exercise*, 2nd ed. Springfield, Ill.: Charles Thomas, 1963.

LOUGHMILLER, CAMPBELL, *Wilderness Road*. Austin, Tex.: University of Texas Press, 1965.

MOUSTAKAS, CLARK, *Psychotherapy with Children*. New York: Ballantine Books, 1970.

OBERTEUFFER, DELBERT, *School Health Education*, 5th ed. New York: Harper & Row, 1972.

RATHBONE, JOSEPHINE, and CAROL LUCAS, *Recreation in Total Rehabilitation*. Springfield, Ill.: Charles Thomas, 1959.

ROSEN, ELIZABETH, *Dance in Psychotherapy*. New York: Bureau of Publications, Columbia University, 1957.

VANNIER, MARYHELEN, *Teaching Health in Elementary Schools*, 2nd ed. Philadelphia: Lea & Febiger, 1974.

WILLGOOSE, CARL, *Health Education in the Elementary School*, 4th ed. Philadelphia: W. B. Saunders, 1974.

8

Other Conditions Requiring Special Services

In addition to the physical and emotional difficulties discussed in the preceding chapters, there are many other kinds of problems that can handicap people and that therefore require special services. These conditions can be caused by disease, accidents, injury, and/or aging. Some are temporary, others permanent. All require some kind of an emotional, physical, and social adjustment. It is important that persons affected by any of these conditions take part in physical activities that will best meet their interests and needs. For some this will be a corrective program, for others, it will be a developmental one.

THE OVERWEIGHT AND UNDERWEIGHT

Three out of every ten American adults are ten to twenty pounds overweight. Most of them are too fat because they are "mouth people"— they eat too much at meals and snack on the wrong kinds of foods throughout the day. Most often their over-eating is caused by loneliness, boredom, and emotional problems. They are physically soft and under-exercised. Obesity among teenagers and children is increasing rapidly. According to medical findings, of every ten persons who are more than ten pounds overweight at 30, only six will live to age 60 and only three to 70. The average life span of the American woman is now around 74.6.[1]

---

[1] Jean Mayor, *Overweight—Causes, Costs and Control* (Englewood Cliffs, N.J.: Prentice-Hall, 1968), pp. 26–29.

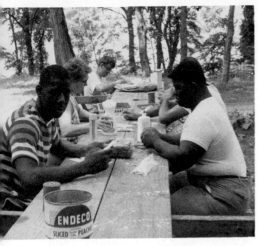

Many of the handicapped are obese. Courtesy of the AAHPER.

Every person has his own body build (somatotype), determined by distribution, muscularity, and linearity. Body typing has been done largely by William Sheldon. From his work, experts now say that the three body types are (as shown in Figure 8–1):

1. *The Endomorph* (a well-padded square box). This type is big, soft, and square and has fat around stomach, hips, neck, and upper arms, but usually has small hands, feet, wrists, and ankles. Such a person moves slowly, is apt to be sluggish, and is often awkward because of excessive bulk.

2. *The Mesomorph* (ideal average, inverted triangle). This type has a well-formed, well-proportioned hard body, arms, and legs. Although the

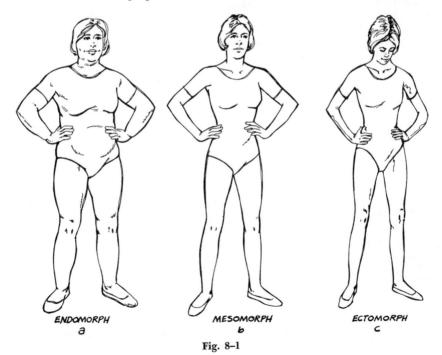

ENDOMORPH
a

MESOMORPH
b

ECTOMORPH
c

Fig. 8–1

mesomorph is somewhat short, he or she has firm muscles, slender waistline, narrow hips topped by broad shoulders. This person tends to be
extrovert, who is good in sports, particularly those that require agility,
strength, balance, and endurance.

3. *The Ectomorph* (frail, thin, and pencil-like.) This type has a long, tall
frame and slim body; underdeveloped muscles; usually constantly trying
to gain weight but nevertheless remains on the frail side. This type tends
to tire easily and lacks energy and sparkle.

Although weight can be lost quickly through crash diets, this practice is both dangerous to one's health and a waste of time.[2] Studies show
that those who go on such diets usually regain all that has been lost plus
ten more pounds within a year. The safest and most lasting weight-loss
programs result in shedding not more than two pounds weekly. Those
who want to lose more than five pounds weekly should do so only with
a physician's guidance. The only true way to lose weight is to reduce
caloric intake and increase physical activity. But strenuous exercise in
itself does not melt pounds away.[3] A person would have to walk 44 miles
or run 129 separate 100-yard dashes in 10 seconds each to lose one pound.
Performing such activities cumulatively is most beneficial. Only self-
discipline in food selection as well as regular exercise will help overweight
people to develop attractive, trim bodies.

A normal person should consume only about 2300 calories daily;
the exact amount depends upon individual size and metabolism. Those
who are underweight according to standardized height and weight tables
need to have a daily diet of 2800 to 3800 calories. Some recommendations for gaining weight include

1. Eating more carbohydrates, fats, and sweets than normal
2. Having an in-between-meal snack at least twice daily (malted milk,
graham crackers with butter and peanut butter, etc.)
3. Drinking a glass of homogenized milk three times daily and at night
before going to bed
4. Reducing the amount of daily physical activity [4]

Adjustment Problems. It is not uncommon for both over- and
underweight people to have deep-seated adjustment problems. However,
they are more common with the former than with those who are too
thin. Many grossly overweight people feel that they are social outcasts;
thus they have marked feelings of rejection and inferiority. Both groups
need to be motivated to correct their way of life, particularly their eating
and exercise patterns. For anyone deviating by ten pounds from a good
weight chart, medical (and sometimes psychotherapeutic) help should
be sought.

---

[2] Theodore Berland, *Rating the Diets* (Santa Monica, Calif.: Rand Publishing
Company, 1974), p. 2.

[3] See Maryhelen Vannier, *A Better Figure for You through Easy Exercise and
Diet* (New York: Association Press, 1965) for specific slenderizing exercises and
suggested diets for all three somatotype groups.

[4] But underweight people, too, need a regular amount of physical activity.

Table 8–1   Desirable Weights for Men and Women According to Height
and Frame, Age 25 and Over

Height in inches in shoes	Weight in pounds (in indoor clothing)		
	Small frame	Medium frame	Large frame
	MEN		
62	112–120	118–129	126–141
63	115–123	121–133	129–144
64	118–126	124–136	132–148
65	121–129	127–139	135–152
66	124–133	130–143	138–156
67	128–137	134–147	142–161
68	132–141	138–152	147–166
69	136–145	142–156	151–170
70	140–150	146–160	155–174
71	144–154	150–165	159–179
72	148–158	154–170	164–184
73	152–162	158–175	168–189
74	156–167	162–180	173–194
75	160–171	167–185	178–199
76	164–175	172–190	182–204
	WOMEN [a]		
58	92–98	96–107	104–119
59	94–101	98–110	106–122
60	96–104	101–113	109–125
61	99–107	104–116	112–128
62	102–110	107–119	115–131
63	105–113	110–122	118–134
64	108–116	113–126	121–138
65	111–119	116–130	125–142
66	114–123	120–135	129–146
67	118–127	124–139	133–150
68	122–131	128–143	137–154
69	126–135	132–147	141–158
70	130–140	136–151	145–163
71	134–144	140–155	149–168
72	138–148	144–159	153–173

Source: Metropolitan Life Insurance Company, *Statistical Bulletin* (November–December 1959), p. 1.

[a] For girls between 18 and 25 deduct 1 pound for each year under 25.

Implications for Physical Education. If one's weight is just right for one's age and height, vigorous daily physical activity will help keep it that way. Remember, though, that the proper kind and amount of exercise (which affects shape) must be accompanied by a well-controlled diet (which affects weight). A total body workout for 20 minutes daily is recommended. It is best to do movements to music; records with a strong 4/4 beat and a peppy tune such as "Hello Dolly" are stimulating; the swing of the music makes one want to move and keep time to it. It is also possible to set a steady rhythmic pattern of your own by counting—for example, bend 1-2-3, back 1-2-3. It is also fun to work out with a partner or a group. One should begin gradually, doing 8 to 10 minutes for the first several days, but time should be increased to 20 or more minutes as soon as possible.

Following are some helpful exercise activities.

Running

Run in place 25 times, starting slowly, picking up speed, and then tapering off. Raise legs high. Increase to 50 times, then to 100, 150, and finally 200.

CONDITIONING EXERCISES

The Twist

Take a stride position, arms out at shoulder height. Twist right on 1, back to place on 2, left on 3. Repeat 25 times.

The Jumping Jack

Take a stride position, hands at side (Figure 8–2). On 1, bring feet together and clasp hands over head. On 2, go back to stride position, hands at sides. Do 25 times.

Knee and Arm Lift

Arms at sides. On 1, swing both arms up, pull in stomach, bend left leg as far as it will go (Figure 8–3). On 2, lower arms to side and bring leg down. On 3 and 4, do the same with arms and right leg. Do 25 times.

EXERCISES FOR THE WAISTLINE

The Star Picker

On tiptoes, stretch high with arms above head. On 1, thrust left arm higher and walk forward (Figure 8–4). On 2, lower it slightly and reach high with right arm while walking forward. Repeat 25 times.

The Sit-Up (modified by bent knees)

Lie on back, knees bent, hands clasped behind head. On 1, sit up, bend to touch right elbow to left knee (Figure 8–5); 2, lie back down;

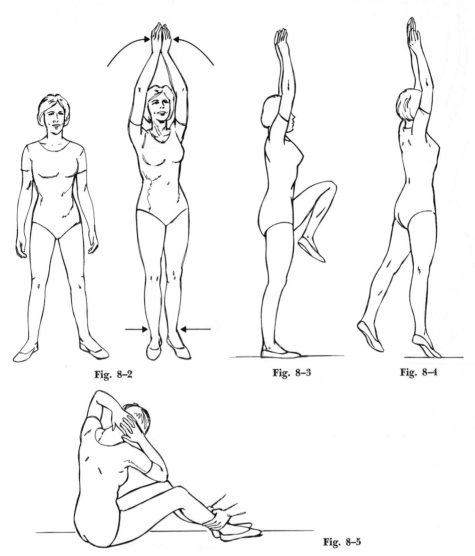

Fig. 8–2   Fig. 8–3   Fig. 8–4

Fig. 8–5

3, sit up, bend, touch left elbow to right knee; 4, lie back down. Do 6 to 8 times.

Jumping Rope

With an individual rope, jump, stretching arms high (Figure 8–6). Gradually increase speed, then taper off. Jump 50 times the first day, 60 the second, 75 the third, and so on.

Long Stretch

Sit with legs extended. On 1, bend to touch toes (Figure 8–7); on 2, return. Do 10 times.

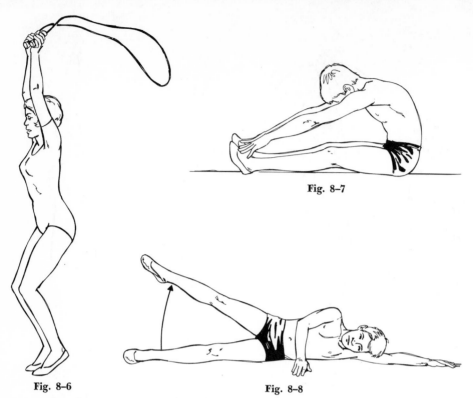

Fig. 8–7

Fig. 8–6

Fig. 8–8

EXERCISES FOR THE HIPS

Scissors Kick

Lie on left side, with head resting on extended left arm. Stretch legs out. On 1, raise right leg up (Figure 8–8); lower it on 2. Do 15 times. Change to right side and repeat.

The Hip Walk

Sit, feet extended. Extend arms to front at shoulder level. On 1, shift weight to left hip and move right hip and leg forward (Figure 8–9a). On 2, do the same for the left hip (Figure 8–9b). Move in rhythm 10 times forward, then 10 times back.

Twister Toe Touch

Take wide stride position with arms extended over head. On 1, twist to touch right hand to left toe; 2, back to place; 3, touch left hand to right toe (Figure 8–10); 4, back to place. Do 15 times.

The Knee-Toe Balance

Stand straight, stomach in, hands on hips. Place instep of left foot on inside of right knee. On counts 1, 2, 3, slowly go up and down on toes (Figure 8–11). Repeat on left foot.

104

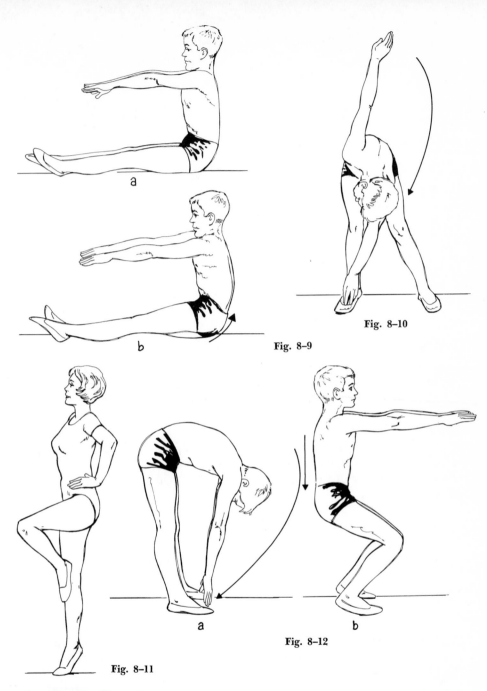

Fig. 8–9

Fig. 8–10

Fig. 8–11

Fig. 8–12

The Dipsy Doodle

With feet together, extend arms in front at shoulder height. On 1, touch feet (Figure 8–12a); 2, return to erect position; 3, bend knees, arms extended to front (Figure 8–12b); 4, back to erect position. Do 20 times, speeding up and then slowing down again.

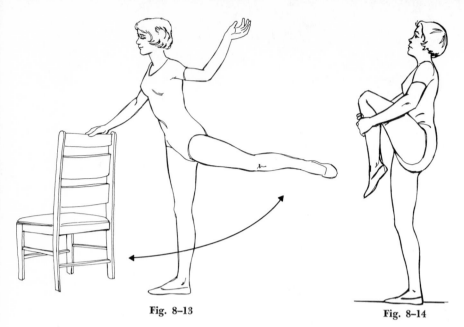

Fig. 8-13   Fig. 8-14

Leg Swings

Standing sideways to chair, hang on to chair for support. Swing the left leg forward in rhythm, back to side (Figure 8–13), and return to front 15 times. Turn, and repeat this pattern with the right leg.

Knee Grasp and Pull

Stand tall. On 1, bend the left knee, grasp the lower leg, and pull toward chest as high as possible (Figure 8–14). On 2, return leg to position. Repeat with right leg on 3 and 4. Do 10 times for each leg.

Tuck and Swing

Stand erect, holding on to a practice bar or chair back. On 1, bend right leg, raise knee to touch chin; on 2, arch back and extend leg straight back as far as possible (Figure 8–15). Do 10 times. Change legs and repeat 10 times.

Leg Circle

Lie face down, chin on back of left hand, right arm straight to the side. Without turning the body, raise straightened right leg, and on counts 1, 2, 3, make 3 circles with it. Reverse positions and repeat with left leg (Figure 8–16). Do 10 times with each leg.

Nip Out and Up

Stand with feet slightly apart. On 1, squat, placing both palms on the floor. On 2, straighten knees and extend legs (Figure 8–17). On 3, return to position. Do 15 times, increasing speed between the sixth and twelfth times, then slowing down.

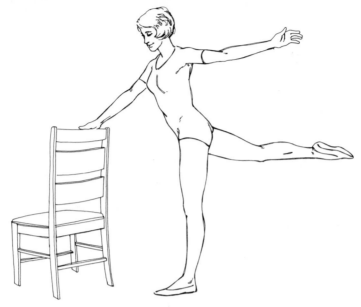

Fig. 8–15

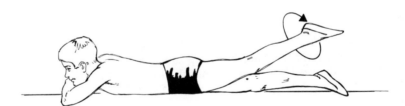

Fig. 8–16

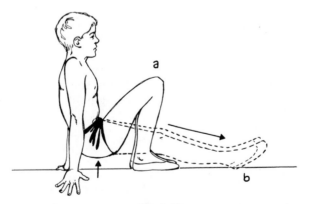

Fig. 8–17

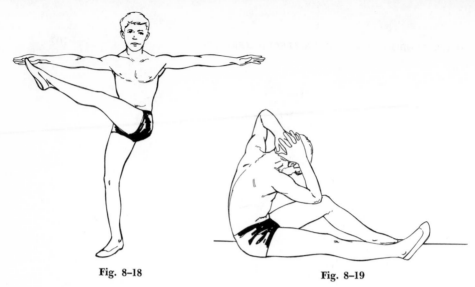

Fig. 8–18   Fig. 8–19

EXERCISES FOR THE WAISTLINE AND HIPS

Hand and Toe Touch

Stand with arms extended to the sides at shoulder level. On 1, swing left leg up to touch right hand, moving the hand as little as possible (Figure 8–18). On 2, return to place. Swing right leg to touch left hand on 3 and 4. Do 10 times.

The Curl-Up

Lie on back, hands clasped behind head, elbows out. On 1, curl trunk forward, bend left knee but keep foot on the floor, and touch right elbow to it (Figure 8–19). On 2, uncurl slowly. Repeat with right knee bent on 3 and 4. Do 10 times. (Have someone hold your feet or place them under heavy furniture.)

The Jackknife

Lie flat on back, back straight, legs together. On 1, curl body up, extend both arms forward and up, and raise both extended legs. On 2, touch ankles (Figure 8–20). On 3, slowly return to position. Do 10 times.

Nose to Knee

On hands and knees, keep arms straight and head up. On 1, curl head in, bringing right knee to touch nose (Figure 8–21). On 2, raise head back and stretch straightened leg back. Do 10 times. Change, bringing left knee to touch nose, and repeat 10 times.

Twist Right and Left

Stand with feet wide apart, arms out to side at shoulder level. Keep the whole of both feet, including heel, on the floor. On 1, twist to the left as far as possible (Figure 8–22). On 2, back to place. On 3, twist right; back to place on 4. Repeat with increased speed, twisting farther each time, for a total of 20 times.

108

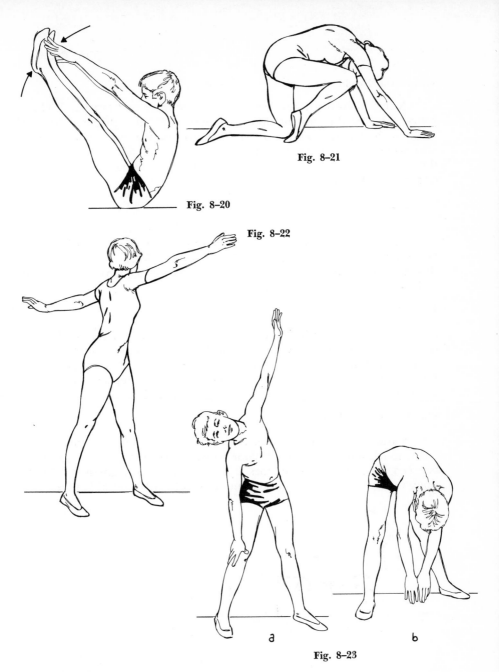

Fig. 8–21

Fig. 8–20

Fig. 8–22

Fig. 8–23

a

b

Eight-Count Stretch

Stand erect, stomach in, hands on hips, feet apart. On 1, stretch arms above head; 2, touch floor between legs with fingers or palms (Figure 8–23a); 3, back to place. On 4, slide right hand as far down right leg as possible, stretch left arm overhead, bend at the waist and stretch on 5, 6, 7. On 8, return to erect position. Repeat series with left arm down leg and right overhead (Figure 8–23b) for counts 5, 6, and 7. Do series 10 times on each side.

Thread the Needle

Kneel, then distribute weight easily on knees and left hand. On 1, bring right shoulder to the floor and push right arm through the arch made by the left arm (Figure 8–24). On 2, withdraw right arm and stretch it briskly overhead. Following movement with head and eyes. Do 10 times, thrusting arm farther on each through and up movement. Change position, using left arm, and repeat 10 times.

Bicycling

Lying on back, bicycle by stretching legs to full extension, toes pointed out. On 1, bend left leg as close to stomach as possible, while extending right leg (Figure 8–25). On 2, reverse. Keep in rhythm, doing this one for the length of a whole record, pushing leg closer to the body and farther away from it each time.

The Stretcher

Lie on stomach with hands clasped behind head. On 1, raise trunk to where waistband or navel touches the floor, and raise straightened legs up 7 to 10 inches from floor (Figure 8–26). Hold for 10 counts, counting 1000-and-1, 1000-and-2, and so on. Relax, rest, and repeat. Avoid overarching the back. A cushion may be used if desired.

The Toe Touch, Centered Back

Stand tall, stomach in, legs comfortably apart and toes turned out. On 1, touch left toes; 2, touch floor between feet. On 3, reach way back between legs; 4, touch right toes (Figure 8–27); 5, straighten up. Do 10 times in slow rhythm, 10 in faster, and taper off with a set of 5 more.

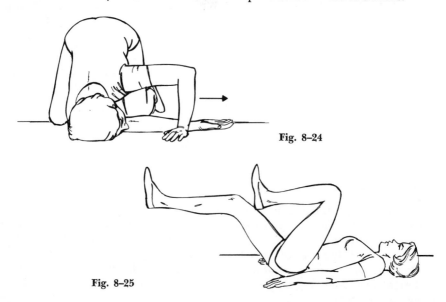

Fig. 8–24

Fig. 8–25

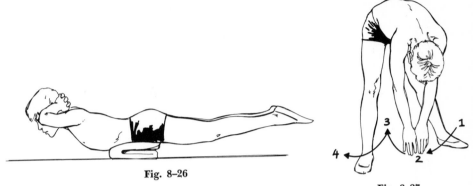

Fig. 8–26

Fig. 8–27

TENSION RELIEVING EXERCISES

One secret of a happy, productive life is found in properly balancing work with play, body tension with body relaxation. Americans live in an increasingly tension-filled world. Some signs of tension are pain at back of the neck, aching shoulders, headaches, burning eyes, and irritability. The tense person is usually touchy, fidgety, and withdrawn. Such tendencies can indeed handicap a person physically and emotionally.

A physical education program can help victims of tension learn how to relax and use their bodies well through a program of exercises. Those who learn this will have a knowledge, a skill, and an appreciation that will probably not only prolong their lives, but also help them to enjoy each day fully.

To relieve tension, exercises like the following are recommended:

The Wilted Daisy

Stand with feet apart. Stretch on tiptoe with both hands over head. Then bend body and shake and wiggle both shoulders, arms, and hands, becoming as limp as possible. Come up slowly on the count of 10. Repeat.

The Head Roll

(*For shoulder tension.*) Stand in a relaxed position. On 1, slowly roll head from front to left shoulder and back on 2. On 3, roll it over right shoulder and back to place on 4 (Figure 8–28). On 5 and 6, slowly roll it all the way around, relaxing neck and shoulder muscles.

Back and Leg Raiser

(*For back tension.*) Lie on floor. On 1, inhale slowly and raise back with body weight supported by head and buttocks (Figure 8–29a). On 2, relax. On 3, inhale and raise right knee to chest, clasping it with both hands (Figure 8–29b). On 4, exhale and extend right knee to floor. On 5 and 6, raise and lower left leg in the same fashion.

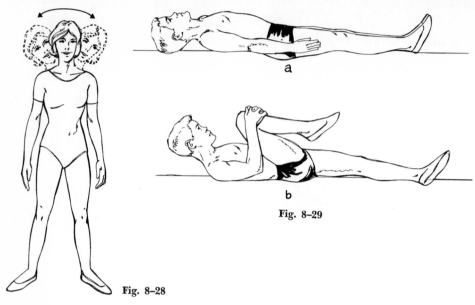

Fig. 8–29

Fig. 8–28

The Tailor Tuck

(For neck tension.) Sit tailor-fashion, with legs crossed. Slowly circle head, keeping shoulders still (Figure 8–30). For variation, sitting in this position, clasp arms behind the head, relax trunk forward; then gradually straighten trunk, starting from lower back. Next curve the back slowly, starting in the neck area.

The Arm Swing

(For tension of the upper back.) Stand, swing left arm forward away from body and back, then both arms, and finally both arms in easy rhythm to music. For variation, raise and lower alternate legs as both arms are swung forward and back (Figure 8–31). This exercise also helps the circulation and flexibility of the back.

The Standing Leg Swing

(For lower back tension.) Stand erect, legs comfortably apart. Swing left leg forward and back in easy rhythm, then right leg. Next, move alternate legs in large circles (Figure 8–32).

The Standing Stretcher

(For back tension.) Stand with feet apart, hands clasped overhead, arms fully extended. Moving left, make a big circle with clasped hands, bending slowly all the way around (Figure 8–33).

The Body Swing

(For general tension.) Holding arms out at shoulder level, swing forward and sideward, stopping sideward swing at the point where tension begins (Figure 8–34, position 1) then back. Swing arms forward, crossing arms in front, sideward.

Next, swing arms forward and backward, using entire body (Figure 8–34, position 2). Flex knees and straighten them on both forward and

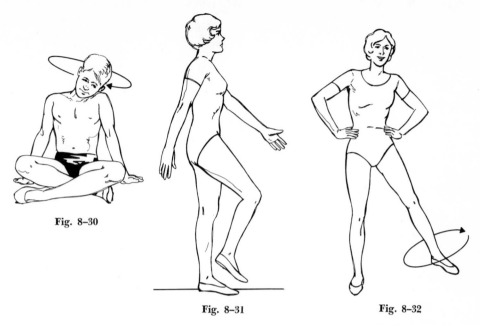

Fig. 8–30

Fig. 8–31

Fig. 8–32

backward swings. Then spread feet far apart, carry swings through the legs (Figure 8–34, position 3).

Next, swing both arms horizontally from side to side. Bend over with body relaxed and start a low swing, gradually straightening up and increasing the perimeter of the swing until the body is erect.

Finally, by experimenting, see how many different swings to music you can do with arms, legs, and body.

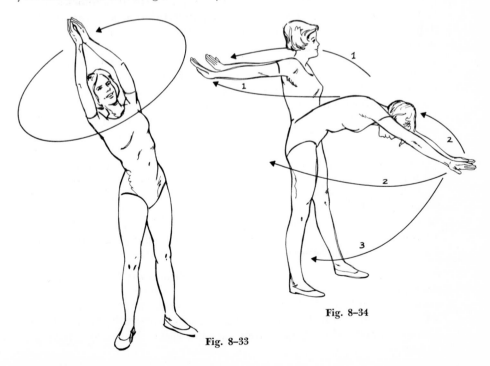

Fig. 8–34

Fig. 8–33

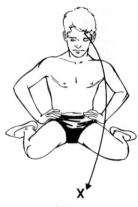

Fig. 8–35

Frog Sitting

(For back and leg tension.) Sit with inside of knee touching floor, legs flexed, hands on hips (Figure 8–35). Inhale, slowly bend forward to touch head to floor in front on count of 1. On 2, slowly exhale and come back to original position.

CHRONIC FATIGUE AND LOWERED VITALITY

People who tire easily or always seem tired and those who are unfit are dragging and drooping their way through life. Boredom, apathy, poor posture, and personality problems exist markedly in this group. As the Greek philosopher, Seneca, has said, "Man does not die, he kills himself."

Fatigue is normal and a part of the rhythm of life, but when it is chronic and coupled with worry, tension, and anxiety, it becomes a major factor in heart, blood vessel, and kidney deterioration and can produce high blood pressure and abnormally early degeneration of various organs of the body. The likelihood of serious heart attacks (our leading cause of death) is also increased. Those who are unfit· are physically many years older than their chronological age; many of the young adults in our society already have middle-aged bodies. Thus fatigue is dangerous, as well as instrumental in preventing a full enjoyment of life.

Physical decline is quickly seen to be the health hazard it really is if you closely observe any heterogeneous group of all ages. As our society becomes more sedentary and affluent, this problem will increase *unless* youth and adults (1) become better motivated to care for their bodies, (2) learn game and sports skills to use in their ever-increasing leisure hours, and (3) play vigorously in order to have fun, release tension, and get a good physical workout. This dangerous trend toward increasing numbers of soft Americans can be reversed, but only when people of all ages become convinced that exercise and vigorous exercise programs truly add life and sparkle to our years.

Adjustment problems. Those who are chronically fatigued and unfit physically usually become group isolates. Some have marked inferiority complexes, and are dull and unattractive to others. In our society, the cultural ideal is for men and women to be physically attractive and healthy. Those who deviate from this ideal may be social rejects and unhappy.

Implications for physical education. Persons suffering from chronic fatigue should know that the best way to *gain* energy and strength is to *spend* energy and strength. It is important, however, to begin slowly, gradually increasing the daily amount of physical activity engaged in.

There are many kinds of quick, revealing phiyiscal fitness tests which can be used to motivate those with chronic fatigue to take part in physical improvement programs.

Below is a questionnaire form for locating tension, fatigue, and other health problems.

Yes   No

___ ___ 1. Do you usually wake up in the morning feeling tired and achy?

___ ___ 2. Do you often fight sleep?

___ ___ 3. Do you often have trouble going to sleep at night?

___ ___ 4. Are you "potty" and/or hippy, with a protruding, sagging abdomen and rear?

___ ___ 5. Are you often "on edge," nervous, or jittery?

___ ___ 6. Is it hard for you to relax during the day?

___ ___ 7. Are you often moody? Worried?

___ ___ 8. Do you have frequent headaches? Twitching face and eyelids?

___ ___ 9. Do you often have indigestion? Bad breath? Constipation?

___ ___ 10. Are you subject to frequent colds? Sore throats? Earaches?

___ ___ 11. Do you have frequent backaches? Joint pains? Aching feet?

___ ___ 12. Does climbing stairs or other moderate exercise leave you breathless?

___ ___ 13. Is it hard for you to stand up or sit up straight for longer than three minutes?

___ ___ 14. Do people generally irritate you?

___ ___ 15. Do you often snack between meals?

___ ___ 16. Do you eat less than three well-balanced meals daily?

___ ___ 17. Are you dissatisfied with your present physical condition?

Boys and girls should be given the President's Council Physical Fitness Test available from the President's Council on Physical Fitness, Washington, D.C. Older youth and adults of both sexes can quickly discover their own fitness level by taking the following test.[5]

1. Score—25 Points   With your shoulders back and your chest expanded, measure the circumference of your chest just below your your armpits. Then measure your waist with your stomach in a relaxed position. Your chest should measure 5 inches more than your waist.

2. Score—10 Points   Sit on the floor with your legs stretching out in front of you, and place an 8-inch-high book upright between your knees. Then, keeping your legs straight and flat on

---

[5] This test is a modification of the Cureton Physical Fitness Test found in Thomas Cureton, *Physical Fitness and Dynamic Health* (New York: Dial Press, 1965), pp. 48–49.

	the floor, bend forward and touch your forehead to the top of the book.
3. Score—10 Points	Stand on your toes, with your heels together, your eyes closed, and your arms fully extended. Stay in this position for 20 seconds without moving your feet or opening your eyes.
4. Score—20 Points	Lie on your back with your hands behind your neck, and raise both legs to a vertical position without bending them. Repeat this 20 times successfully.
5. Score—15 Points	Support your body stretched sideways on one hand (with your arm held straight) and the outside of one foot. Place your other hand on your hip. Raise and lower your upper leg to a horizontal position 25 times without bending either knee.
6. Score—25 Points	Lying flat on your stomach, face down, with your fingers laced behind your neck and your feet remaining on the floor, raise your chin until it is 18 inches off the floor and hold this position for 10 counts.
7. Score—10 Points	From a kneeling position, with the bottoms of your feet facing up and your arms stretched forward from the shoulders, swing arms up, jump to a standing balanced position without moving either foot to maintain balance.
8. Score—20 Points	Lie on your back with your hands behind your neck, your legs flexed. Do 25 sit-ups without resting.
9. Score—10 Points	Do a standing broad jump. The length of your jump should be approximately equal to your height.
10. Score—50 Points	Run in place for 60 seconds, lifting your feet at least 4 inches from the floor. Then take three deep breaths. Then hold your breath for thirty seconds.

Less than 100 points on this test indicates an urgent need for an intensive conditioning and physical activities program.

ANEMIA

Anemia is caused by conditions that affect the red blood cells. It is a symptom, not a disease, and is a signal that something is wrong. One of the most common causes is loss of blood—for example, from excessive menstrual blood flow or frequent pregnancy—and from a lack of iron in the diet.

Symptoms of anemia are fatigue, weakness, shortness of breath, and tingling in the hands and feet. If anemia is found to exist, a physician can determine from a blood test what type of anemia it is and give proper treatment.

Chlorosis anemia occurs in many young women during puberty and is characterized by less hemoglobin in the blood corpuscles than is normal. *Pernicious anemia* is due to a decrease in the number of red corpuscles and can be serious. *Iron-deficiency anemia* is common among adult women in our society; *aplastic anemia,* wherein fatty marrow replaces red bone marrow, is relatively uncommon, for it results from atomic fallout, excessive radiation, and radioactive isotopes.

Adjustment Problems. Those who are anemic are chronically fatigued, listless, and often unstable. They drag through each day, receiving little pleasure from their activities. Anemic children tend to be too sheltered by their parents and have resulting emotional problems of hypochondria and self-centeredness. Both they and anemic adults are generally watchers rather than doers.

Implications for Physical Education. Because exercise, and especially that done out-of-doors, helps in the production of red blood corpuscles and increased blood circulation, the anemic should be encouraged to take part in those games and sports which are more fun to play outside (such as tether ball for children or golf for adults). However, they should also dress properly, for anemic people are most vulnerable to respiratory infections.

The best type of physical and recreational programs for people with this problem depends upon which kind of anemia they have. The recommendations of a physician are also important. Great care must be taken to begin slowly, gradually increasing the amounts and kinds of activity. Efforts should be centered around helping those afflicted to gain strength, endurance, and improved coordination and motor skills. Increased physical activity must prove to be beneficial rather than detrimental. Exercises that can improve posture and general appearance should also be stressed.

MENSTRUAL PAIN

Although today only a minority of girls and women suffer from menstrual pain (dysmenorrhea), the right types of exercise in sufficient amounts can work wonders. Those with severe pain should consult a physician (preferably a gynecologist).

Most girls and women suffering from cramps preceding or during menstruation have weak pelvic floor muscles supporting the visceral organs. Strengthening these muscles daily through specific exercises not only relieves menstrual difficulties but usually leads to ease in childbirth later. It is important to know, however, that performing a few of the following exercises will *not* help unless they are done daily for 15 to 30 minutes over an extended period of time. The following exercises are recommended for menstrual pain.

The Daisy Droop

Stand straight (Figure 8–36a), slump over, and tighten stomach muscles on counts 1–2–3 (Figure 8–36b). On 4–5–6, return to erect position; on 7–8, return to slump position with stomach muscles tightened; on count 9–10, relax, return to erect position. Repeat 10 times.

Foot-Feet Patty Cake

Lie on back with arms bent out and up from sides. Keep legs straight and raise them 3 inches from the floor. Bring feet together and apart in patty-cake fashion 25 times (Figure 8–37).

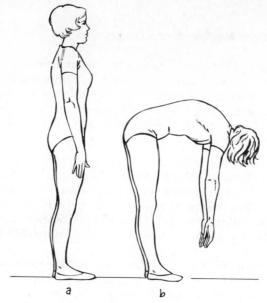

Fig. 8–36

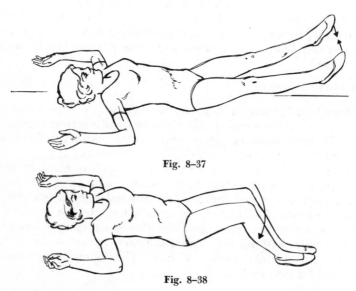

Fig. 8–37

Fig. 8–38

The Bent-Knee Twist

Lie on back as described in the previous exercise. Flex knees, tighten stomach muscles, and keep shoulders flat on the floor while turning lower body and legs over to the right, then to the left (Figure 8–38). Repeat 25 times.

The Camel Hump

With weight on hands and knees, arch back on counts 1–2–3–4, and tighten stomach muscles (Figure 8–39a). Relax on 5–6–7–8 (Figure 8–39b); repeat 10 times.

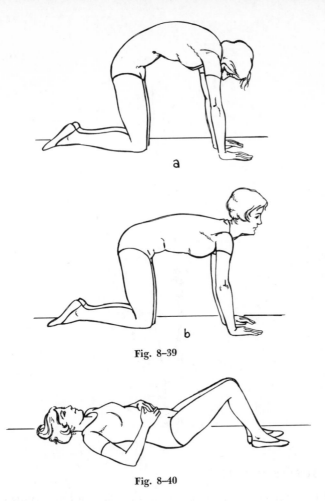

a

b

Fig. 8–39

Fig. 8–40

The Grasshopper

Kneel supporting body weight on hands and knees to suspend internal organs while in this unnatural position for three minutes. Stand erect. Repeat 10 times.

The Mosher Exercise

This exercise is a "pumping" exercise; hands become the pumping power. Lie on back and flex knees, keeping feet flat on the floor. Place both hands on stomach, take a deep breath, and push down with both hands (Figure 8–40). Exhale and relax. Repeat 10 times daily.

The Golub Exercise

Stand with body and arms in full extension, and with knees locked (Figure 8–41). On count 1, twist, turn body to right; on count 2, bring fully extended left arm across your body to touch your outer right heel and fully extend your right arm back for balance. Repeat on other side. On 3, swing both fully extended arms forward, and at the same time, kick left leg backward. On 4, return. Repeat arm swing on 4 and then kick back with the right leg. Repeat 20 times.

119

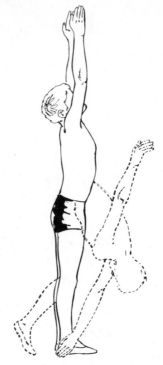

Fig. 8–41

DIABETES MELLITUS

It is estimated that there are around one million known diabetics in the United States—one person in every 150 is a diabetic. Although 10 percent of these victims are children, more than two-thirds are over 40 years of age. Thanks to the discovery of insulin by Dr. Frederick Banting and Dr. Charles Best, many diabetics live nearly normal lives.

Diabetes is an inherited disease caused by the malfunctioning of the insulin-secreting cells in the pancreas; the body is thereby robbed of a major source of energy. Mild cases can be controlled by diet and exercise; more serious cases are controlled by daily injections or oral consumption of insulin. The disease is incurable but controllable. The diabetic must watch his diet carefully and, if he has a serious case, must be constantly alert to avoid going into a state of unconsciousness or shock. Regulated exercise is important in the control of diabetes, but it must be the right kind and amount as determined by a physician. Diabetics are especially subject to boils and other types of infections. The feet must be carefully kept from injury and infection, and the diabetic needs to have special instructions as to their care, including directions for treating corns and calluses, how to avoid blisters and athletes' foot, and even for cutting nails.

Exercise decreases the need for insulin, helps to control weight (obesity and diabetes are related), and contributes to physical vigor. Although the diabetic can take part in most of the same kinds of activities as the normal person, the instructor should be alert to signs of fatigue. Candy or fruit should be available in case of insulin shock.

EPILEPSY

The term *epilepsy*, coming from the Greek word for "seizure," is used to describe what happens when brain cells discharge too much electrical (nervous) energy. The patient loses consciousness and has no muscle control during most types of seizure. Although most doctors do not believe that epilepsy is inherited, it is thought that a tendency toward the disease may be inherited. Generally epilepsy does not get worse with age, and often those who have seizures early in life do not have them as frequently or intensely as they grow older. Epilepsy is a symptom; it cannot cause mental retardation or inanity. Most people who have it are of normal or above-normal intelligence. Many famous persons have had it, including Julius Caesar, Alfred the Great, Lord Byron, Swinburne, de Maupassant, Paganini, and Van Gogh.

Epilepsy is much more common than most people realize. About one in every 100 persons—approximately 2 million Americans—have it. Because of much prejudice and misunderstanding about this malady, it is difficult to get accurate information concerning the actual number of persons afflicted by it. However, it is known that there were at least twice as many persons suffering from it than from cancer in the United States in 1969, and that as many people have it as diabetes. It is estimated that there are as many as 25 million epileptics throughout the world and that there are 1,500,000 epileptics in the United States.[6]

Epilepsy is caused by anything that affects the metabolism of the brain cells. It can be caused by faulty brain development before birth, brain injury during birth, head injuries, brain tumors, faulty blood circulation, or certain metabolic disorders. In epilepsy, irritative injuries to the brain vary in location. There are a dozen different types. Often the severity of a seizure depends upon which part of the brain has been irritated. The symptoms vary from seizures lasting only a few seconds (*Petit Mal* or "Little Sickness") to gross twitching convulsions in which the person becomes unconscious (*Grand Mal* or "Big Sickness").

A Jacksonian seizure starts on one side of the body and gradually spreads. Another type is characterized by one sudden jerk of the head, legs, or trunk. In another kind, symptoms are dizziness, pain, sweating, heart palpitation, and vomiting. In another type, psychomotor epilepsy, the victim goes into a trance and becomes almost completely unaware of what is going on. Sometimes in a seizure, the person has violent temper

---

[6] Richard Kraus, *Therapeutic Recreation* (Philadelphia: W. B. Saunders, 1973), p. 7.

tantrums, stares, mumbles, and jerks at his clothes. In still another type, one attack follows right after another and the patient has to be hospitalized for rapidly repeating convulsions and high fever. Many new medications obtainable from a physician can reduce the number and severity of seizures. The electroencephalograph, an instrument for measuring electrical impulses of the brain, is of great diagnostic value.

Adjustment Problems. Those who are epileptic usually attend regular school if their attacks are controlled by drugs. Should a seizure occur in school hours, others should be helped to understand the disease. During a Grand Mal seizure, the victim first becomes unconscious and thrashes around, and sleepiness or extreme fatigue follows. Afterward, the person is unaware of what he did or of any danger he was in during the seizure. Something soft, such as a tightly rolled scarf, might be placed between the victim's teeth during an attack. Furniture or objects that might be struck during the convulsion should be moved.

Implications for Physical Education. It is imperative that all leaders know of the presence of an epileptic in a group and what to do should an attack occur. All those having this malady should be carefully supervised. Because they rarely have seizures while playing, group participation should be stressed, as well as activities which require concentration. The controlled epileptic can benefit from physical conditioning and taking part in competition that requires concentration and controlled body movements. Swimming, rope climbing, and other activities in which they might be in danger if an attack occurs must be avoided.

Suggested physical activities for epileptics include:

Archery
Bait and fly casting
Hiking and camping
Games of low organization
Table games such as checkers, chess, etc.
Table tennis
Social, folk, and square dancing
Skating
Weight lifting
Wrestling

CONVALESCENCE

Studies show that physical and recreation activities for those who are ill or recovering from surgery can speed up that recovery. Most of our hospitals for the armed forces now provide such therapeutic programs for those recovering from injuries received while in combat duty. Modified and adapted physical activities which can help produce total body fitness are now being used widely with remarkable success in both schools and hospitals.

Until recently, school physical education programs were largely for the well and healthy; little provision was made for those who returned to school following major illness or an accident. Fortunately, the practice of excusing such students from taking part in physical activities is rapidly disappearing. In our better schools today, convalescing students are increasingly placed in an adaptive physical education program in which they are greatly aided in developing strength, endurance, and vitality.

Many physically active persons who become bedridden or hospitalized develop emotional disturbances, anxieties, and fears, all of which retard recovery. Many think that they are sicker than they actually are, become discouraged from having to be waited on, and feel that they are a burden to their family. Recreational and physical education programs, in both schools and hospitals, do much to boost morale and help speed the return to normal life.

The Hospital Program. Patients in hospitals include those who are:

1. Soon to be able to go home
2. Ambulatory cases
3. No longer solely confined to bed but able to have restricted amounts of physical activity
4. Confined to bed but able to take part in some light physical exercises and activity
5. Too ill to take part in any kind of activities, physical or recreational

Most large hospitals have a department of physical medicine, a physical and/or occupational therapist, and recreational specialists. All such personnel are a part of the rehabilitation team headed by a physician and composed of specialists and volunteers. There may be a gymnasium, game room, or recreation center in the hospital as well as mobile carts with exercise equipment that are wheeled into the patients' rooms. These contain weights, balls, and elastic exercisers. Such carts also carry books and magazines, tables games and puzzles, arts and craft materials.

Mild or strenous exercises for those lying supine in bed, those able to sit up in bed, young children, those confined to wheelchairs, or those on crutches should be given by specialists in therapeutic recreation as prescribed by a physician. Ball and target throw games, modified croquet, shufflebord, square dancing, and weight lifting are among the activities recommended.

Program for Those Returning to Schools. It is important that students returning to school following an illness be placed in an adaptive physical education class. Most of them are weak and have a low level of strength and endurance. Each, knowing when he is too tired to continue, should determine when rest periods should be taken. However, the teacher should encourage each student to play for a slightly longer time period, for the only way to *gain* strength is to *spend* strength. In cases where there has been a specific injury, such as a neck whiplash, great care must be taken to strengthen rather than further damage the injured area. Consequently, each student's physician or the school doctor should prescribe the specific exercises to be used.

The adaptive physical education class should be kept small, and individual attention should be given by the teacher to each student. Suggested activities include:

Archery	Deck tennis
Billiards	Horseshoes
Bowling	Shuffleboard
Box hockey	Swimming
Dancing	Table tennis
Darts	Volleyball

CARDIOVASCULAR INVOLVEMENTS

Over half of all deaths in our country are due to heart disease. Those having heart disorders of a serious nature below the age of 25 are the victims of congenital heart abnormalities or rheumatic fever, which now affect more than 500,000 children. Although some of these children can attend school only part of the time, many must be taught at home by a visiting teacher.

Cardiovascular disorders include rheumatic fever, congenital heart involvement, hypertensive heart disease, coronary heart disease, and cerebrovascular disease. It is imperative that the physical educator especially, as well as other teachers, know which students have heart trouble and the seriousness of each condition. Rheumatic fever and congenital heart disease affect more children than adults, although many of the latter have heart damage of which they may or may not be aware as a result of rheumatic fever, which has symptoms similar to those of the common cold. Teachers and parents need to be on the lookout for children who seem listless, fail to gain weight, have frequent colds and sore throats, and complain that their legs and joints ache (too often erroneously thought to be "growing pains"). Often the disease recurs (in 50 to 70 percent of cases), and almost always its victims break out in a rash and have high fever and pain. The brain can become affected as a result by what is called St. Vitus dance, and the heart valves can be damaged.

The American Heart Association has classified those with cardiopathic and circulatory disturbances as follows:

Organic Heart Disease

    Class I —Patients with organic disease, but able to carry on physical activity

    Class II —Patients with organic disease, but able to carry on either slightly or greatly limited physical activity

    Class III—Patients with organic disease who cannot have any physical activity and must remain in bed

Possible and Potential Heart Disease

    Class I —Patients with *possible* heart disease, not believed to be due to organic heart disease

Class II—Patients with *potential* heart disease—patients without circulatory disease whom it is advisable to follow because of a history of etiological factors which might cause disease

Adjustment Problems. Often those with a diagnosed heart malfunction become extremely anxious and shun physical exercise. Those born with a congenital heart defect tend to be better adjusted and less cautious than those who develop it later in life. An alarming number of adults who suddenly have heart attacks panic and become almost complete invalids. Others, thinking their life is almost over, start burning the candle at both ends, thus shortening their lives even further.

All persons of school age having heart involvements should have a periodic physical examination, receive guidance and counseling, be provided with transportation if necessary, receive vocational guidance, be placed properly in classes from which they will receive the greatest benefit, and have frequent rest periods throughout the school day.

Implications for Physical Education. Cardiac students should be placed in the physical education class best suited to their needs as determined by a physician, for the program must be composed of activities within the physical capacity level of each student. The daily instructional period should include short activities followed by longer periods of rest. Under no circumstances should cardiac students engage in competitive sports. Elementary children should be more closely supervised than those on the secondary level. For them, suggested activities are:

Movement exploration
Rhythms and dance
Croquet
Table games
Tag and "it" games
Leadup games to sports such as Newcomb for volleyball
Jacks
Small table billiards

Bowling with rubber balls
Table tennis
Bicycling
Relays
Simple games
Darts and quoits
Story plays
Miniature golf

On the secondary or adult levels, suggested activities include:

Archery
Circle games
Bag punching
Camping and campcraft activities
Fishing, hiking, hunting
Juggling
Horseshoes
Badminton and tennis doubles
Canoeing and sailing

Roller and ice skating
Rope spinning
Swimming and water games
Ping pong
Shuffleboard
Paddle tennis
Ring toss
Volleyball
Pitch and putt golf
Social and folk dancing

HERNIA

A hernia is an abnormal protrusion of an organ or other body part through the containing wall of its cavity. Most hernias are found in the abdomen but they may occur in the chest as well as in other areas. A noncongenital form results from strain, weight lifting, operation, or muscular weakening. Congenital hernias exist at birth and are surgically corrected as soon as possible. Hernia is more prevalent in males and found more frequently in those who are greatly overweight.

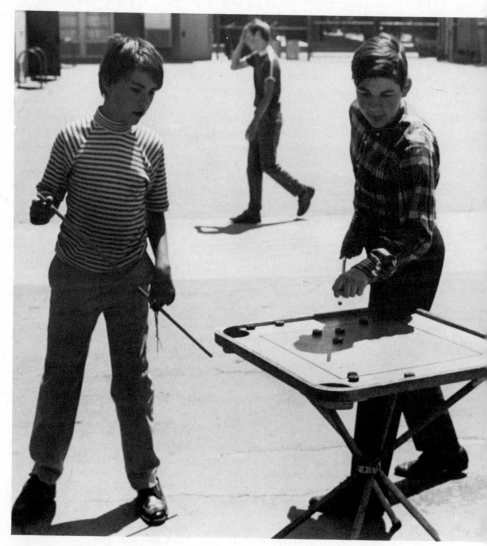

Asthmatic children can enjoy learning to play a modified game of billiards and develop hand-eye coordination at the same time. Courtesy of the Los Angeles Public Schools.

Those who have hernia should avoid all physical activities (such as weight lifting or boxing) that could cause increased strain in the affected area and those sports (such as football and soccer) that could cause injury to that area. Rope climbing, gymnastics, tumbling, and activities requiring excessive running, such as track and field activities, must be avoided. Activities most suited to hernia victims include golf, table tennis, billiards, fly and bait casting, bowling, and swimming.

Exercises that will strengthen the muscles of the abdominal wall should be done daily as prescribed by a physician or physical therapist. This exercise period might well be followed by games or other physical activities which bring challenge and pleasure to those having hernias.

ALLERGIES

A hypersensitivity or allergy is a body condition in which there is an exaggerated reaction to certain kinds of foreign substances. Some persons are allergic to certain foods, such as eggs or strawberries; others have reactions to ragweed or other plants; while still others may be allergic to certain animals, such as cats or horses.

An allergy can cause stomach upsets, rash, hives and sneezing, watery eyes, and other symptoms of the common cold. Treatment includes medication and the avoidance of the causative agent. Physical activities for those who are allergic to pollens and dust should be held indoors, and the area should be as dust-free as possible. Progressive developmental activities (such as learning to play table tennis and proceeding to advanced badminton) are suggested.

SUGGESTED READINGS

BRALEY, WILLIAM, *Daily Sensorimotor Training Activities*. Freeport, N.Y.: Educational Activities, 1969.

CRATTY, BRYANT, *Movement Behavior and Motor Learning*. Philadelphia: Lea & Febiger, 1969.

———, *Developmental Sequences of Perceptual-Motor Tasks*. Freeport, N.Y.: Educational Activities, 1967.

DELACOTO, CARL, *The Diagnosis and Treatment of Speech Reading Problems*. Springfield, Ill.: Charles Thomas, 1964.

KRUSEN, F. H., F. J. KITLKE, and P. M. ELLWOOD, eds., *Handbook of Physical Medicine and Rehabilitation*. Philadelphia: W. B. Saunders, 1965.

LOWMAN, CHARLES, *Postural Fitness*. Philadelphia: Lea & Febiger, 1960.

MATHEWS, DONALD, ROBERT KRUSE, and VIRINIA SHAW, *The Science of Physical Education for Handicapped Children*. New York: Harper & Row, 1962.

RADLER, D. H., and NEWELL KAPHART, *Success Through Play*. New York: Harper & Row, 1960.

RUSK, HAROLD, *Rehabilitation Medicine*. St. Louis: C. V. Mosby, 1965.

SCHOENBOHM, W. B., *Planning and Operating Facilities for Crippled Children.* Springfield, Ill.: Charles Thomas, 1962.

VANNIER, MARYHELEN, *Body Conditioning, Figure and Weight Control for Women.* Belmont, Cal.: Wadsworth Press, 1973.

VODOLA, THOMAS, *Individualized Physical Education Program for the Handicapped Child.* Englewood Cliffs, N.J.: Prentice-Hall, 1973.

WILLIAMS, HARRIET, and VIRGINIA BEANE, "A Comparison of Selected Behavior of Identical Twins, One Blind from Birth," *Journal of Motor Behavior,* 1, No. 4 (December 1969), 259–73.

THE PROGRAM

Never check the actions of the child; follow him and watch to prevent any serious accidents, but do not even remove obstacles which he would learn to avoid by tumbling over a few times. Teach him to jump rope, to swing weights, to raise his body by his arms, and to mingle as far as possible in the rough sports of the older boys. Do not be apprehensive of his safety. If you should see him climbing in the branches of a tree, be assured he is less likely to fall than if he had perfect vision. Do not too much regard bumps on the forehead, rough scratches, or bloody noses; even these may have their good influences. At worst, they affect only the bark and not the system like the rust of inaction.

Dr. Samuel Gridley Howe, patriarch in the field of education of the visually handicapped

9

Program Planning and Evaluation

Because some students have special health and safety problems, these should be carefully taken into account when planning any physical educational or recreational program. Successful activities programs for the handicapped within public schools, other institutions (hospitals, specialized schools, etc.), and the community depend on the use of procedure, methods of classifying people and assigning them to specialized activity regimens, and so forth. This chapter will deal with some of the ways of implementing effective physical activities programs.

PROGRAM PLANNING

To be of value, physical activities programs must be more than mere entertainment or time-fillers. They should be carefully planned with definite objectives in mind so that the participants as well as leaders know what is to be accomplished, what the main purpose is, and how each activity relates to the total program. Likewise, they should be primarily concerned with helping others find physical fitness, joy, beauty, and meaning in life. This is particularly relevant when dealing with handicapped people.

The leader must care deeply about people, their present welfare, their future, and the destiny of humanity. The program is the magic wand with which people can be touched and receive lasting benefit. The leader's primary role is to help each participant grow as a unique individual and become a contributor of positive gains in our society. His or her primary concern should be to teach people through activities and not merely to direct programs. What a person learns about human relations and life through the program offerings is of great importance.

Principles of Program Planning

Principles are truths or basic beliefs that can be action guidelines. As professional leaders of integrity, those in charge of planning activities for the handicapped should strive to provide a program that has value, is of the highest quality, and will benefit all those taking part in it. There are times, however, when program changes must be made and compromises devised. As long as the leader can operate upon such basic principles as "the greatest good for the greatest number," or "the community recreation program should be for all the people all of the time, instead of just for children in the summer," he is on the right track.

One authority said:

> Expediency and compromise of principles are always fraught with danger of personal integrity. One may give way on a minor principle in order to gain a major one, or one may accept a present defeat in view of a promise of a later victory. The ultimate test, however, is a professional rather than a personal advantage, a cause served rather than a profit gained.[1]

Every physical education and recreation program should

1. Provide equality of opportunity for all, regardless of sex, age, race, or religion
2. Be based upon the age, sex, needs, capabilities, and interests of all individual participants
3. Serve co-recreational and fellowship needs
4. Provide for family participation both as a unit and separately for all individuals within it
5. Be planned in light of the desired goals and objectives sought by the sponsoring group, the instructor, and each individual participant
6. Be devised to make the best possible use of all available community facilities and other resources, available equipment, and the leader's various leadership skills
7. Be wide enough in scope to be of present and future value to the individual, community, state, and nation
8. Be one which every person can engage in safely and one which will lead to improved health and total fitness (physical, mental, and emotional)
9. Be planned for the betterment of social and moral behavior
10. Be flexible, with provisions made for instructor-group planning and modification
11. Be planned to develop degrees of skill among the beginners, intermediates, and advanced participants in each activity

---

[1] Jesse Feiring Williams, *The Principles of Physical Education*, 8th ed. (Philadelphia: W. B. Saunders, 1964), p. 24.

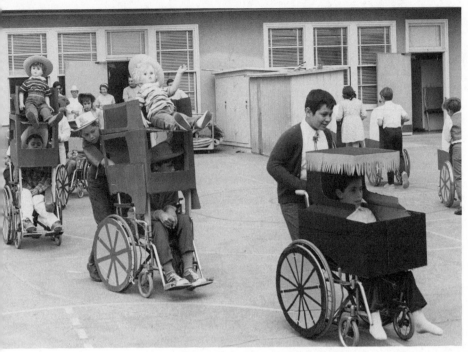

All children love being in a parade! Courtesy of the Los Angeles Public Schools.

12. Provide outlets for self-expression and creativity
13. Include carefully planned activities for the ill, handicapped, and aged in such places as prisons, hospitals, and institutions
14. Be well-balanced with both active and passive activities
15. Help build recreation patterns and hobbies of lasting value
16. Be modified and improved upon as the results of continuous evaluation by all who plan, take part in, and administer it

Influences on Program Planning

The success of any learning program for the disabled depends upon the ability of those in charge of it to (1) draw up daily, weekly, monthly, and seasonal program offerings according to established goals and objectives and (2) carry these plans out successfully. In smaller community centers or playgrounds where only one or two people are in charge of the entire program, ideas can be gathered from many sources. These include the individuals or groups to be served, other physical activities specialists, periodicals, and books. Specialists, especially, welcome the opportunity to educate others in the nature, purpose, scope, and value of programs. Some of the best ideas for program improvement, however, often come from those who take part in it. Leader-group planning helps others to gain democratic leadership skills and an understanding of their importance, increases interest and personal identification in the program, helps others gain increased responsibility for their own choices and actions, and aids in the development of stronger leader-group rapport, with resulting friendlier group relationships.

133

Interests of the Participants. All programs, to be of value, must be based upon the interest, needs, and abilities of the group. When involved in group planning, the poorest approach is to ask the group members what they want to do, for the majority will cling to old favorites, rebel against anything new, or will follow the suggestions made by the most persuasive person in the group. The use of an interest questionnaire has merit for discovering the real interests of each individual.

After these results have been tabulated, the leader and group-selected representatives will be better able to plan a program that will reach the needs and interests of the majority. For such planning the group should be composed of the leader and not more than five or less than three persons. Minor matters, such as how to choose teams for tournament play and voting procedures, can be settled by the entire group. This concept of leading with the assistance of elected subleaders is important. It can be used most successfully and is a learning laboratory for democracy.

Learning the real interests of any group or of any individual is fundamental to good planning. The role of the leader is to recognize the development level of a person and to guide him or her to learn new and challenging activities and make richer discoveries.

Age. Every age group has its own unique characteristics, interests, needs, and favorite things to do. However, grouping of different ages can be used successfully, too. The majority within such classifications will fit generalized characteristics. Recognition of the interests of each developing group as well as members' readiness or ability to learn sports and games is of paramount importance.

Planning for adults is often harder than planning for children, because many adults are more afraid to lose face among their peers. Likewise, it is more difficult to help grown-ups gain movement mastery, such as in dancing, unless they have had experiences in earlier childhood in rhythmical response and moving to rhythm. Adults also tend to be more routinized than youth in their recreational patterns and often are less eager to do something entirely new. Adults playing in sports and games can be classified largely according to age and sex for some activities, and grouped together for others. Youngsters and older people, for example, can belong to the same hobby clubs or take part together in activities such as music, crafts, nature, and dramatics.

Sex Differences. Recent studies show that differences between the sexes in ability to excel in sports are not as great as once believed. Girls and boys differ in play interest largely because of cultural conditioning, which begins soon after birth. Little boys have traditionally been given balls to play with; girls given dolls. And each tend to copy in play the habits and roles of the adult male or female. Actually, women have the same potential to excel in sports and games as males; yet throughout history boys and men have had a greater opportunity to take part in sports and have thus gained more mastery and interest in them.

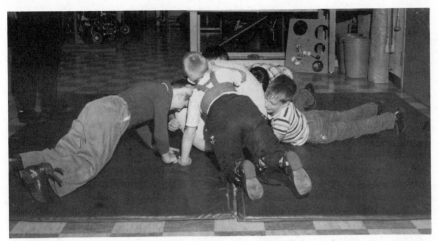

Boys will be boys before they learn to become men in our highly competitive society. Courtesy of the AAHPER.

It is often best, because of variance in acquired interest and strength, to plan highly competitive sports events separately within each sex group for boys and girls who have reached puberty. Competition for girls and women should include events that stress skill and form, such as tennis or synchronized swimming. Competition for boys and men should include sports that call for strength and speed and are more rugged, such as weight lifting, handball, or tackle football. During adulthood, co-recreational activities such as mixed volleyball, bowling, and swimming are popular, as are music, crafts, dancing, and camping.

Older adults seemingly favor co-recreational activities such as dancing, cards, or dramatics. Men have traditionally enjoyed such craft activities as woodworking or metalwork; women have preferred activities that centered around the household acts, such as interior decorating or sewing. However, even this pattern is changing.

Facilities. Ideally, the program should determine the facilities. Unfortunately, few leaders are fortunate enough to be able to start a program from scratch and then plan a building or other type of facility in which to conduct it. Rather, most leaders are stuck with what facility is available and must modify their program accordingly.

Leadership is the key to the successful recreation program. It is far more important than any impressive facility. Ingenious leaders learn to utilize fully available community resources. Some conduct early-morning bowling classes or leagues in commercial alleys. Others conduct a splendid program in schools during the summer months or during the evenings. Still others use store parking lots for Sunday-afternoon or evening programs. "Where there is a will, there is a way," and any leader truly believing in this old saying will find facilities in which to conduct a well-planned program.

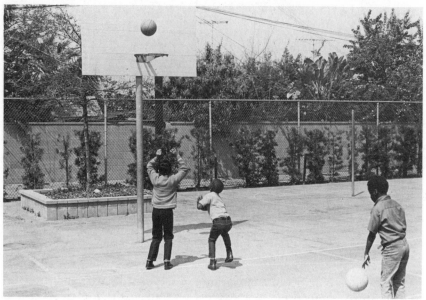

The recreation area should provide both indoor and outdoor play space for both supervised and free-play activities. Courtesy of the Los Angeles Public Schools.

Multiple-purpose tennis courts can also be used for handball, roller and ice skating, dancing, volleyball, basketball, goal shooting, and shuffleboard. The use of lighting alone will bring many participants to a recreational facility, thus reducing the cost for a program when determined by the number of people served.

Time. Industrial recreation specialists have learned to provide activities before and after work hours as well as during the noon hour. Schools have been doing this for a long time through their intramural competitions, club programs, and recess activities. Many communities now have bowling alleys and other facilities open all night in order to accommodate people who work at odd hours.

Special events, such as pet shows and parades, an old settler's reunion, Santa Claus visit, or a local fair add variety to any planned year-round recreation program. Seasonal sports activities, whether they be swimming and baseball for the summer months or ice skating and skiing in the winter, help to stimulate and maintain interest among all age groups. Timeliness is good program planning. Also important is a sense of timing. The wise leader is one who recognizes that some events are more successful when planned on a short-term basis: for example, a model airplane club; others, such as a tennis class for beginners, are more successful when carried on for several weeks. The type of activity, coupled with the skill required to master it, is a major determining factor in all program planning.

Size of Group. Although it is always impressive to have a large number of people taking part in any recreational or educational activity, what happens to each individual within the group is vastly more important than how large the group is. Many activities are best for not more than ten people, especially in such things as hobby clubs or beginning golf or swimming—and more particularly in classes for handicapped people.

The size of the group should also determine how it can be serviced best. A baseball or bowling league may be organized on a citywide basis. Some large municipal recreation departments, such as the one in Dallas, Texas, have one physical educator whose primary job is to set up all league and tournament play. Because many sports bring greater satisfaction to individual players when they provide for competition and/or teamwork, with scheduled times to play and practice, the development of league play is highly recommended.

The Scope of the Program

In its totality, a well-balanced physical activities program will consist of:

Creative-cultural activities
Social activities
Camping and outing activities
Physical activities including sports and games
Service activities
Special events

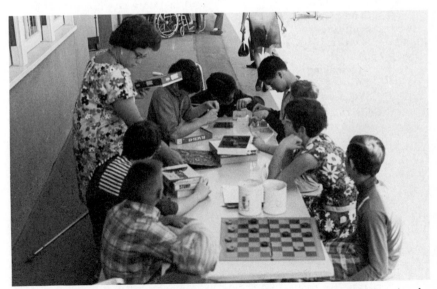

Table games and crafts can be enjoyed by all age groups. Courtesy of the Los Angeles Public Schools.

Under the separate parts are often found the following items:

Creative-Cultural Activities

Arts and crafts
  Basket making
  Beadcraft
  Block printing
  Bookbinding
  Cabinet making
  Carving
  Ceramics
  Costume design
  Drawing
  Dyeing and coloring
  Embroidery
  Etching
  Finger painting
  Knitting
  Leather work
  Metal craft
  Model airplanes
  Painting
  Paper folding
  Photography
  Pottery
  Reed and raffia
  Rug making
  Sand painting
  Sculpture
  Sketching
  Tincraft
  Toy making
  Weaving
  Wood carving
Collecting
  Antiques
  Books
  Buttons
  Coins
  Dolls
  Furniture
  Glassware
  Guns
  Indian craft
  Paintings
  Ships
  Stamps
Dancing
  Acrobatic

    Ballet
    Clog
    Creative
    Tap
Drama
    Charades
    Festivals
    Impersonations
    Informal dramatics
    Making scenery
    Marionettes
    Mask making
    Masquerades
    Minstrel shows
    Movies
    One-act plays
    Pageants
    Pantomimes
    Parades
    Play reading
    Punch and Judy shows
    Puppetry
    State craft
    Story plays
    Storytelling
    Vaudeville acts
Mental
    Book clubs
    Debates
    Discussion groups
    Forums
    Guessing games
    Lectures
    Mental games
    Public speaking
    Puzzles
    Reading
    Study groups
    Television watching
    Tricks
Musical
    Bands
    Barbershop quartets
    Glee clubs
    Orchestras
    Solo instruments

Social Activities

Banquets
Basket suppers
Beach parties
Card games
   Bridge
   Canasta
   Hearts
   Pinochle
   Pit
   Poker
Carnivals
Conversation
Dancing
   Folk
   Social
   Square
Dinners
Family reunions
Parties
   Birthday

   Block
   Costume
   Seasonal
Pencil and paper games
Potluck suppers
Scavenger hunts
Table games
   Anagrams
   Caroms
   Checkers
   Chess
   Crokinole
   Dominoes
   Monopoly
   Parchesi
   Pickup sticks
   Picnicking
Treasure hunts
Visiting

Camping and Outing Activities

Bait and fly casting
Barbecues
Boating
Camping
Canoeing
Corn roasts
Clambakes
Crafts from native materials
Fish fries
Gardening
Hiking
Horseback riding
Hostelling
Making nature trails
Mountain climbing
Nature study
   Astronomy
   Bee culture
   Birdhouse building
   Caring for pets
   Collecting

   Animals
   Birds
   Bugs
   Flowers
   Minerals
   Mosses
   Rocks
   Snakes
   Trees
Rifle shooting
Skeet shooting
Skiing
   Snowshoeing
   Snow tracking
Tobogganing
Trap shooting
Trapping
Visiting zoos
Walking
Wiener roasts

Physical Activities

Archery
Badminton

Baseball
Bicycling

Box hockey
Boxing
Bowling
Croquet
Darts
Deck tennis
Driving
Fencing
Field hockey
Football
Golf
Handball
Horseshoes
Ice skating
Jacks
Kite flying
Lacrosse
Ping pong

Roller skating
Rope skipping
Rope spinning
Shinny
Shuffleboard
Soccer
Softball
Speedball
Squash
Stunts
Tennis
Track and field
Tumbling
Volleyball
Wading
Water polo
Weight lifting
Wrestling

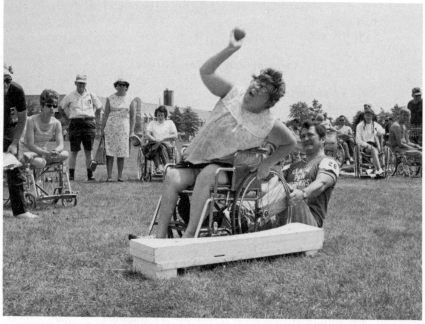

A recreation program might be planned to include a track and field meet. Courtesy of the National Wheelchair Athletic Association.

Creative Ideas in Programming

Albert Einstein once wrote that he considered ingenuity to be greater than knowledge. Certainly it is true that the most successful leaders in any recreation or physical education program are highly creative. They can see program possibilities and needed materials for carrying them out in discarded junk, waste products made of paper, wood, or wires, and even discarded automobile tires. Some are smart enough to capitalize upon the cultural backgrounds of certain communities or subgroups within them. The Spanish Cultural Night, held yearly in Albuquerque, New Mexico, grew out of such an idea. The Tulip Festival, sponsored jointly by the Atlanta Recreation Department and the Atlanta Tulip Study Club, annually includes over 600 folk dancers in Dutch-patterned costumes adding color and rhythm to a program in which a beauty queen and her court are honored. Thousands of people in Atlanta enjoy watching this entertaining program. Such citywide programs can lead to increased participation in other program activities sponsored by the community recreation department and foster good publicity and public relations.

Community service activities help people feel that they have something of value to give to others. Many youth-serving organizations, such as Scouts, the Campfire Girls, or YMCA groups receive assistance from volunteer parents, who help set up programs and summer camps for the handicapped. Such worthwhile activities yield far more return than just saving money, for they help others gain a feeling for and identification with others.

Such suggested planned volunteer activities will provide outlets for those who enjoy working with people. However, it is recommended that the professional leader who sponsors such a program have several orientation meetings, in-service briefings, and a final evaluation period with all taking part in the program. The purpose of such a program, it should be stressed, is to help people learn *how* to help themselves. As in the Peace Corps, only qualified volunteer leaders should be used; those who are to work directly with the handicapped must be particularly carefully screened.

EVALUATION OF THE PROGRAM

Evaluation is a method of appraising, measuring, and checking progress. It is a way of finding out where you are in relationship to where you want to go. Properly used, evaluative techniques tell you more about (1) pupil progress, including health status, behavior, and reaction to the program and fellow classmates; (2) the teacher's ability to teach and reach individuals as well as a class group successfully; (3) strengths and weaknesses of the program; and (4) better ways to explain to parents, professional colleagues, school administrators, and the general public how physical activities are helping the handicapped. To be most effective, evaluation should be continuous. It should be done by all who participate in and/or are affected by the program. Finally, it must be concerned both with end products and the means with which to reach these ends. Such evaluation is of great importance, particularly when one is working with the handicapped.

Methods of evaluating pupil progress and the physical activities program include the use of:

Skill tests
Written tests of knowledge, attitudes, and habits
Observation
Checklists
Rating scales
Interviews
Case studies
Diaries
Parental conferences
Self-appraisals
Group discussions
Questionnaires
Social development tests
Physical examinations
Personality inventories
Health records
Surveys

The teacher most frequently uses observation as a method of evaluation. But this tool is subjective and must be used with skill in order to be of value. The various objective evaluative techniques require careful, planned, step-by-step procedures. For example, the effective administration of tests includes:

Advance preparation
    Selecting the test
    Gaining an understanding of a test to be used and how it is to be administered
    Obtaining necessary equipment and facilities
    Preparing score cards for individuals by class roll or squads
Administering the test
    Done by the teacher entirely
    By paired groups with one-half scoring, the other taking the test, in reverse order
    By squads, by the squad leader or other trained class assistants
    Using the station-to-station method, rotating groups to certain testing areas
    Using any combination mentioned above
Devising scoring methods, recording results by the teachers, assistants, squad leaders, or paired partners
Duties during the test
    Providing a warm-up period
    Demonstrating each item
    Motivating each pupil to do his best
    Taking safety precautions when necessary

Duties following the test
  Grading the tests
  Converting raw scores to percentages on a scoring table
  Comparing results with norms and constructing profiles
  Informing pupils of the results
  Using the results for classification, guidance, research grading, and motivation
  Evaluating one's effectiveness as a teacher and noting what areas need to be changed or reviewed

The following are the specific purposes of physical education testing for children: [2]

1. To determine the status of boys and girls in relation to fundamental human values amenable to improvement through physical education activities and methods
2. To determine the status of boys and girls in relation to basic body traits which affect physical performances
3. To classify pupils according to their abilities in physical activities
4. To measure the results of instruction in physical and motor skill activities

Evaluation of Health Status and Physical Growth

Although annual physical examinations are advisable for all children, some school authorities believe that there are four times when periodic examinations are essential: when the child enters first grade, during the middle elementary experience, at the beginning of adolescence (during the junior high school years), and before leaving the senior high school. Throughout a child's school experience, he or she can also be referred to the school physician or a specialist because of a teacher's observation or as the result of a screening test. The physical examination for children as well as adults was discussed briefly in an early chapter; however, it is worth repeating that for evaluative purposes, a careful record should be kept of all findings, for this appraisal is not an end to itself, but rather a means of helping each person gain better health.

Ideally, all children should be weighed and measured each month in the elementary school, and an accurate record should be kept for each pupil. Although weight norms are available from insurance companies, each teacher should use these only to compare the records of each pupil in relationship to those of many children of the same age and grade in school. It is important for the teacher to know that such things as inherited maturational tendencies, emotional problems, and illness can all affect growth.

---

2 Harrison Clarke and Franklin Haar, *Health and Physical Education for the Elementary School Classroom Teacher* (Englewood Cliffs, N.J.: Prentice-Hall, 1964), p. 69.

Adults should also be weighed periodically and careful records kept on weight gain and/or loss, for either is an indication that the body is not being cared for as it should be.

The NEA–AMA Physical Growth Record is often used in elementary schools for recording a child's growth pattern over several years.[3] Such a record is valuable in noting growth patterns and deviations. Other recommended screening tests include: [4]

For Vision
   The Massachusetts Vision Test
   The Holmgren Wool Test for color-blindness
For Hearing
   Discrete Frequency Audiometer Test
   The Watch Tick
   The Massachusetts Group Pure Tone Test
   The Coin Click Test
For Posture and Body Mechanics
   The New York State Posture Test
   The Kraus-Weber Refined Posture Test
   The Kelly Foot Pain Test
   The Footprint Angle

Evaluation of Social Growth and Behavior

A continous record of behavior is also essential in evaluating individuals, progress, or lack of it. The following chart can be used for recording and studying pupil behavior.

Behavior Sheet

Name _____ School Year _____ Age _____
Physical Activity Class _____

Does the person:	Frequently	Seldom	Never
Take an active part in playing group activities?	_____	_____	_____
Take an active part in playing?	_____	_____	_____
Express himself confidently?	_____	_____	_____
Accept criticisms and suggestions from his peers?	_____	_____	_____
Accept criticisms and suggestions from adults?	_____	_____	_____
Take turns with others?	_____	_____	_____
Show above-average leadership ability?	_____	_____	_____
Have many consistent friends?	_____	_____	_____

---

[3] See Carl Willgoose, *Health in the Elementary Schools*, 4th ed. (Philadelphia: W. B. Saunders, 1974), p. 51.

[4] Complete directions for giving all these screen tests can be found in Carl Willgoose, *Evaluation in Health Education and Physical Education* (New York: McGraw-Hill, 1961).

	Frequently	Seldom	Never
Change friends often?	_____	_____	_____
Play fairly?	_____	_____	_____
Seem interested in improving skills or learning new ones?	_____	_____	_____
Assume responsibility without being reminded or threatened?	_____	_____	_____
Seem happy and well-adjusted?	_____	_____	_____

Comments

1. _____
2. _____
3. _____
4. _____
5. _____

Areas in which the person needs help:

1. _____
2. _____
3. _____
4. _____
5. _____

What I will do to help him help himself:

1. _____
2. _____
3. _____
4. _____
5. _____

Signed _____

Date _____

Such records can be of great help to the teacher in gaining insight regarding pupils.

The use of a sociogram is also recommended.[5] Here children are asked to write the names of class members they would like on their team. By this device, the teacher can identify group isolates, rejects, and leaders.

Evaluation of Motor Skills and Physical Fitness

Many tests have been developed to measure motor ability, motor intelligence, and physical fitness. Almost all measure strength and endurance, innate coordination, speed, reaction time, balance, kinesthesis,

---

[5] A good way to do a sociogram is to ask any group to imagine having a Christmas party and asking each to write the names of any two from the group he would ask. Through this method, the leader can discover who in the group is the most popular and more isolated by his peers.

flexibility, agility, and body explosive power. Suggested tests for doing so on the elementary level are: [6]

Brace Motor Ability Test
Vertical Jump Test
Burpee Test
Carpenter Motor Ability Test
Iowa Brace Test
Kraus-Weber Floor-Touch Test for Flexibility
AAHPER Youth Fitness Test
New York State Physical Fitness Test
Oregon Motor Fitness Test
Amateur Athletic Union Junior Physical Fitness Test [7]
President's Council on Physical Fitness Test [8]
Washington Motor Fitness Test [9]
California Physical Performance Test [10]
The Carpenter General Motor Capacity Tests [11]
Latchaw Motor Achievement Test [12]

Evaluation of Knowledge and Attitudes

Written tests include objective questions which require short answers, longer essay answers to general questions, rating scales, and problem situation questions which require short but well-thought-out answers.

Written tests are of the greatest value when the teacher fully understands what it is she wants to test, knows what to do with the results, and has found the best measuring instruments for these purposes.

TRUE-FALSE TESTS

Educators contend that these are the poorest and weakest kind of objective test questions to use. Pupils tend to read meaning into each statement; few can tell the difference between a correct or incorrect state-

---

[6] See Clarke's or McCloy's book listed in the bibliography for complete directions for giving the first six tests.

[7] Directions for this fitness test are available from the Amateur Athletic Union, 233 Broadway, New York, N.Y. 10007.

[8] Available from U.S. Government Printing Office, Washington, D.C., 1961.

[9] Available from Dr. Glenn Kirchner, Eastern Washington State College, Cheney, Washington 99004.

[10] Available from the Bureau of Health Education, Physical Education and Recreation, California State Department of Education, Sacramento, California 95814.

[11] Arleen Carpenter, "Measuring General Motor Capacity and General Motor Achievement in the First Three Grades," *Research Quarterly*, 13 (December 1942), 444.

[12] Marjorie Latchaw, "Motor Achievement," *Research Quarterly*, 25 (December 1954), 429.

ment or can resist mentally tinkering with it; few things are really completely true or entirely false.

All true and false statements should be short and simple. They should avoid using the words "never" or "always." Have the pupils use the symbols (+) or (0) instead of (T) or (F), because those unsure of the answer often deliberately make the marks hard to tell apart. Other ways to score the test include encircling T if the statement is entirely true, or F if it is only partly true, or blocking out X in the first colum if the sentence is correct and encircling it if the second one is wrong. In the first grade, or with the mentally retarded, have the children draw a face with the mouth turned down if the statement is false, or with mouth turned up if it is true.

Example: Write + if the statement is true, 0 if it is false.

Hit-Pin Baseball

0	1. Five Indian clubs are used in this game.
0	2. Each run scores two points.
+	3. The ball, when kicked fair, must be sent to first, second, third, home base, in this order.
0	4. The pitcher may throw the ball to the kicker.
+	5. The kicker is out on the third strike.

MULTIPLE-CHOICE TESTS

These questions should be short, clearly written, and not copied word for word from a textbook. Care must be taken not to make answers obvious, or not to set a pattern through which the correct answers can easily be found.

MATCHING TESTS

These questions are best for measuring the mastery of "where," "when," and "who" types of information. They do not develop the ability to interpret or express oneself. The responses to the matched items should be placed alphabetically or numerically in the right-hand column. Blank spaces should be provided in the left column before each item to be matched. There should be at least two more answers in the right column than in the left.

Example: Match the items in the left column with those in the right. Some answers in the latter may be used twice.

Tennis

C	1. A score of no points or 0 points	A. Deuce
A	2. Score of 40–40	B. Winner of two out of three sets
B	3. Match	C. Love
		D. 40

D	4. Players score with three points	E. Ad in or ad out
E	5. Next score after 40–40	F. 15–15
F	6. Each player has 1 point	G. Winner of three out of five sets
		H. 40–50
		I. 10–10

FILL-IN BLANKS

The chief drawback to this type of examination is that students have difficulty filling in blanks in the exact words the teacher expects; thus, they are often given the benefit of the doubt or cause the teacher to become irritated and more exacting as she continues to grade the paper. Also, it is time-consuming to grade such questions. One advantage to using this type of test is that the pupil is not guided to the answer

Example: Write the correct answer in the blank provided for it below.

Square Dance

1. The   (head)   couple usually stands with backs to the caller.
2. The lady usually is on the gentleman's   (right)   side.
3. Honor your partner means to   (bow to your partner)   .
4. The last line of the call "all jump up and never come down" is   (swing your honey round and round)   .
5. Three running steps followed by a hop is done in a   (schottische)   .

ESSAY QUESTIONS

These questions provide pupils with opportunities to compose complete sentences and whole paragraphs and to think through problems carefully. Their drawback is that they are time-consuming to read and difficult to grade. However, such answered questions help teachers to gain additional insights concerning their pupils and their unique personal problems. Examples of good essay questions are:

1. What are the values of being physically educated?
2. How have your own recreational patterns been improved as a result of taking this class?
3. What is your definition of good sportsmanship?

RATING SCALES

Pupils enjoy rating and evaluating their own work or habits in school. The best scales for doing so are those devised by the class. Teachers can help children benefit from this type of experience by personal follow-up conferences with each child.

Example: Pupil's personal evaluation of daily health habits.

	Always	Frequently	Seldom	Never
1. I exercise every day.	___	___	___	___
2. I eat fruits and vegetables every day.	___	___	___	___
3. I drink a quart of milk daily.	___	___	___	___
4. I eat between meals.	___	___	___	___
5. I get enough sleep and rest so that I feel good.	___	___	___	___

Evaluation by the Pupils

People within learning situations should be given many opportunities to evaluate what progress they have made in relationship to the goals set individually and by the group. (Needless to say, we are referring throughout to handicapped, as well as normal people.) Teachers should appraise progress with the learners, as well as being continually observant of students' reactions to what they are doing, and their attitudes toward the teacher, the class, themselves, and life in general. Time should be taken frequently to discuss these reactions. Problems that have arisen should be discussed. And future goals and plans need to be determined by learners and teachers-leaders together.

Deeper insight and a clearer understanding of the group as a whole, as well as of the feelings of the class toward the teacher, can be gained by having each pupil write on an unsigned paper answers to the following type of questions at the end of a semester or a major class project.

1. Did you enjoy this experience? Why?
2. List the new things you have learned in order of importance to you.
3. What activities have you done away from school that you learned here?
4. What person do you most admire in our class? Why?
5. How could you be like this person, if you wanted to?
6. What did you hope to do or learn that you did not?
7. What pupil do you think improved the most? In what ways?
8. Are the pupils here learning to be good citizens? In what ways?

Much information can also be gained by having pupils complete statements that show inner feelings, fears, or thoughts. Suggested questions include the following:

1. My greatest fear when I am in this class is that I _____

2. I think my ability in sports and games is _____

3. I dislike _____ because _____

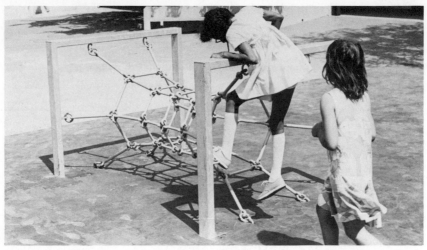

The real test of any learning experience is what the learner *does* when away from the teacher. Courtesy of the Los Angeles Public Schools.

4. I would like to be just like _____ because _____

5. I _____ this class, because here I _____

    There is great educational value in having pupils submit sample objective test questions with their correct answers. They can also benefit from grading each other's papers in class as the teacher reads the correct answers. Every real educator will find ways to utilize any time spent in evaluating progress to its utmost, and will make good use of test findings in order to improve as an effective leader.

    The pupils may feel freer to speak truthfully if they are asked to write suggestions for class improvement and turn them in unsigned. Another method is to have each pupil fill in a checklist such as the following:

Pupil Evaluation Sheet

	Always	Frequently	Seldom	Never
Do you enjoy classes in physical activities?	____	____	____	____
Do you feel as though you are getting enough individual attention in learning to do new things?	____	____	____	____
Do you play the activities learned in class after school and during your leisure time?	____	____	____	____
Do you feel as though your class gives you enough opportunities to get to know a number of activities and people?	____	____	____	____
Do you feel as though you have gained in skills?	____	____	____	____

List the things you like most about this physical activities class.

1. _____
2. _____
3. _____

List the things you like least about this physical activities class.

1. _____
2. _____

How do you think this class could be made better?

1. _____
2. _____

Teacher Evaluation

Every teacher should take a frequent realistic look at herself and her work. A suggested evaluation sheet for doing so follows:

	Always	Frequently	Seldom	Never
1. I like teaching.	____	____	____	____
2. I enjoy my students and try to understand them.	____	____	____	____
3. I am democratic.	____	____	____	____
4. I feel inadequately prepared to do my job well.	____	____	____	____
5. I make the best use of student leadership.	____	____	____	____
6. I make the best use of facilities and equipment.	____	____	____	____
7. I have my own teaching objectives clearly in mind for each class.	____	____	____	____
8. I have my objectives clearly in mind for the development of each unique individual student.	____	____	____	____
9. I plan my work ahead.	____	____	____	____
10. I teach something new every class period.	____	____	____	____
11. I am cognizant of carryover values in what I am teaching.	____	____	____	____
12. I give skill and written tests periodically and use them to evaluate my work.	____	____	____	____
13. I feel that the students admire me.	____	____	____	____
14. I have discipline trouble.	____	____	____	____

	Always	Frequently	Seldom	Never
15. I try to cooperate with my administrators.	_____	_____	_____	_____
16. I feel the other teachers respect me.	_____	_____	_____	_____
17. I join professional organizations, attend their meetings, and read their periodical literature.	_____	_____	_____	_____
18. I feel that I am making a real contribution to my professional field.	_____	_____	_____	_____

Things I should do to improve myself as a teacher are:

a. _____   e. _____
b. _____   f. _____
c. _____   g. _____
d. _____   h. _____

                                                    Date _____

My progress on this so far has been:

a. _____   c. _____
b. _____   d. _____

                                                    Date _____

Evaluation with Supervisors

The school administrator should be aware of the work accomplished by all teachers during the school year. He or she should visit each teacher regularly and offer suggestions for improvement. Such a person must often be the go-between for teachers and the general public. By observing classes in physical activities and by reading reports submitted by the teacher, he can gain insight into the program.

The task of teaching also includes that of educational diagnosis. The teacher's analysis of each class should include consideration of what the students have accomplished during their class period, learning problems that were evident with the entire group as well as with individuals, and possible solutions for learning stumbling blocks.

Tests are necessary tools for evaluating learning. Each unit of work within a physical activities program should include a written and a skill test. These should be easily administered and not be too time-consuming to grade or record. Not more than two class periods should be taken for these tests.

Evaluation of the School Program

Three major areas of a school physical activities program should be evaluated periodically: the effectiveness of the teacher conducting the program, the facilities, and the program content. Such an evaluation could be made by a visiting team of physical activities experts, the teachers involved in the program, and the school administrator. Periodic meetings should be held to review the results of such evaluations, and specific plans should be drawn up to eliminate existing weaknesses and add viable improvements. Consultants should be brought in to work with the teaching staff to improve offerings, if necessary.

An evaluative form such as the following might be used by those reviewing the program in its entirety:

Program Evaluative Form

A. *The Instructional Staff*   *Yes*   *No*

1. Is the teacher a college graduate with a major in elementary education? _____ _____
2. Has the teacher had at least one three-hour course in special or adapted physical education within the past five years? _____ _____
3. Has the teacher attended any clinics or workshops in special physical education within the past three years? _____ _____
4. Is the classroom teacher assisted by a physical activities specialist in planning and conducting the program? _____ _____
5. Can the teacher demonstrate a wide variety of movement skills or sport skills correctly? _____ _____
6. Can he/she diagnose faulty movement patterns and correct movement imperfections? _____ _____
7. Does the teacher follow a graded course of study in adapted physical education? _____ _____

B. *The Facilities*

OUTDOOR

1. Is the outdoor play space a safe place for students to play? _____ _____
2. Is the area fenced? _____ _____
3. Are all playing areas well-marked, drained, and free of debris? _____ _____
4. Are the youngest children assigned a place to play that is (a) furthest away from the oldest children's area; (b) near the school building? _____ _____
5. Is there sand, tanbark, or sawdust under all apparatus to protect pupils from injury? _____ _____
6. Are all pieces of equipment thoroughly checked periodically for safety purposes? _____ _____
7. Are all pupils taught the safest way to use all outdoor equipment? _____ _____
8. Are the pupils well-supervised before and after school when playing, and during noon hour? _____ _____

INDOOR

1. Is there a well-lighted, well-ventilated gymnasium used for both instructional and free-play purposes? _____ _____
2. Is the gymnasium a safe place for students at active play? _____ _____
3. Are all court and boundary lines well-marked? _____ _____

4. Is there adequate storage space for all equipment and supplies?   _____   _____

5. Can all needed equipment be easily and quickly moved to all teaching areas?   _____   _____

C. *The Program*

1. Do teachers periodically help plan and revise a printed course of study?   _____   _____

2. Are the teachers and pupils aware of the objectives of the program in its entirety and of each daily lesson therein?   _____   _____

3. Does the program contain a variety of activities under the broad headings of aquatics, rhythmic activities, movement exploration, stunts and tumbling, elementary gymnastics, simple games, lead-up games to team sports, and outdoor education?   _____   _____

4. Does the instructional program really produce skill learning in a variety of activities or is it merely a supervised play period?   _____   _____

5. Are there adequate established ways in which the program can be evaluated by the teacher, the pupils, and the school administration?   _____   _____

6. Is the school program correlated with the school health and safety programs?   _____   _____

7. Does the program meet the amount of time designated for daily class instruction in physical education set by state law?   _____   _____

According to the above findings, the weaknesses of this physical education program seem to be:

a. _____
b. _____
c. _____
d. _____

Things that should be done to improve this program are:

a. _____
b. _____
c. _____
d. _____

SUGGESTED READINGS

ADAMS, RONALD, ALFRED DANIEL, and LEE RULLMAN, *Games, Sports and Exercises for the Physically Handicapped.* Philadelphia: Lea & Febiger, 1972.

American Association of School Administrators, Council of Chief State School Officers, and National Association of Secondary-School Principals: *Testing, Testing, Testing.* Washington, D.C.: National Education Association, 1962.

CHAPMAN, FREDERICH, *Recreation Activities For The Handicapped.* New York: Ronald Press, 1960.

CLARKE, H. H., and D. H. CLARKE, *Developmental and Adapted Physical Education*. Englewood Cliffs, N.J.: Prentice-Hall, 1963.

Current and past issues of *Parks and Recreation Magazine, The Journal of Health, Physical Education and Recreation,* and *The Instructor*.

Department of the Interior, Bureau of Outdoor Recreation, *Outdoor Recreation Planning for the Handicapped* (April 1967).

KRAUS, RICHARD, *Recreation Today, Program Planning and Leadership*. New York: Appleton-Century-Crofts, 1966.

KRAUS, RICHARD, and JOSEPH CURTIS, *Creative Administration in Recreation and Parks*. St. Louis: C. V. Mosby, 1973.

LATCHAW, MARJORIE, and CAMILLE BROWN, *The Evaluation Process in Health Education, Physical Education and Recreation*. Englewood Cliffs, N.J.: Prentice-Hall, 1967.

LEWIS, GERTRUDE, *The Evaluation of Teaching*. Washington, D.C.: National Education Association, 1966.

National Easter Seal Society for Crippled Children and Adults, "Evaluation of Program Effectiveness and Community Needs," *Rehabilitation Literature,* 31, No. 1 (January 1970).

⸻, "Evaluation of Rehabilitation Programs," *Rehabilitation Literature,* 32, No. 3 (March 1971).

⸻, "Forecast for the Future: Research and Public Support," *Rehabilitation Literature,* 31, No. 5 (May 1970).

⸻, "New Dimensions in Rehabilitation Services," *Rehabilitation Literature,* 31, No. 6 (June 1970).

⸻, "Prejudice and Rehabilitation of the Socially Handicapped," *Rehabilitation Literature,* 32, No. 1 (January 1971).

⸻, "Recreation Counseling," *Rehabilitation Literature,* 31, No. 8 (August 1970).

POMEROY, JANET, *Recreation for the Handicapped*. New York: Macmillan, 1964.

SCOTT, M. GLADYS, and ESTHER FRENCH, *Measurement and Evaluation in Physical Education*. St. Louis, C. V. Mosby, 1960.

SMITHELLS, PHILIP, and PETER CAMERON, *Principles of Evaluation in Physical Education*. New York: Harper and Brothers, 1962.

VAN DER SMISSEN, BETTY, *Evaluation and Self-Study of Public Recreation and Park Agencies: A Guide with Standards and Evaluative Criteria*. Arlington, Va.: National Recreation and Park Association.

VANNIER, MARYHELEN, *Recreation Leadership*, 3rd ed. Philadelphia: Lea & Febiger, 1975.

WHEELER, RUTH and AGNES HOLEY, *Physical Education for the Handicapped*. Philadelphia: Lea & Febiger, 1970.

WILLIAMS, ARTHUR, *Recreation for the Senior Years*. New York: Association Press, 1962.

10

Facilities, Equipment, Supplies, and Transportation

FACILITIES

Generally speaking, the handicapped need the same kind of facilities as the normal. Regardless of the type of facilities available for the handicapped, they should be modified when necessary so that the handicapped people will need a minimum of assistance to enter, leave, or move around in a given space with a maximum degree of independence. Those on crutches or in wheelchairs need the greatest amount of modification of facilities and equipment. Some recommended provisions are:

1. Permanent ramps installed at entrances and exits
2. Handrails and parallel bars for those who are on crutches
3. Smooth nonslippery nature trails, hallways, and rooms
4. Lowered phones and drinking fountains for those in wheelchairs
5. Widened gates, doors to toilet facilities, and exits for those in wheelchairs
6. For sand and water play, specially built tables at heights functional for both wheelchair and ambulatory participants
7. Permanent tables and stools of varying heights installed for quiet games and eating purposes
8. Eyebolts with safety belt attachments for the most severely disabled so that they can stand without falling while doing crafts or when playing table games
9. Such things as lowered basketball hoops so that wheelchair victims can fully enjoy this type of activity

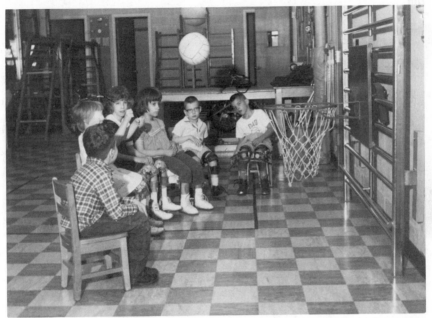

Facilities and equipment often have to be modified when teaching the handicapped. Courtesy of the AAHPER.

10. Box-style swings with a protective guardrail for the most severely handicapped

11. Blacktopping of all playground areas and near buildings for added protection and safety purposes

12. A pool with a wide deck and a slip-proof surface; water level flush with pool deck in order to allow for easy pool entrance

13. Steps with handrails built with short risers and wide steps leading into the pool; ramp with parallel bars so persons unsteady on their feet can enter the pool by themselves

14. Specially built carts to wheel the severely handicapped into the water or a Hoyer lift with which a person can be lifted from a wheelchair and lowered into the water and placed in the sleeve in the concrete at the water's edge [1]

15. Ramps with protective rails for fishing in a lake or pond

16. Pontoon boats riding at deck height out of the water so those in wheelchairs can take part in boating

17. Guide ropes for track and field events, nature trail walking, and other activities for the blind

18. Food service areas with tables that are about 30″ from floor to the underside of table; also, cafeteria self-service areas widened for those in wheelchairs

---

[1] Write to the National Recreation and Park Association for more information about the Hoyer lift, or order the pamphlet that describes it, *Outdoor Recreation Planning for the Handicapped,* from the Superintendent of Documents, U.S. Government Printing Office, Washington, D.C. 20402.

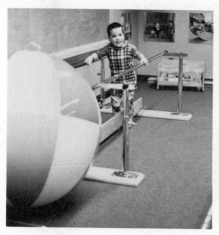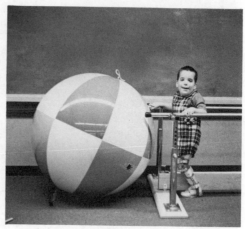

Parallel bars are used in teaching crippled children to walk. Courtesy of the Richardson, Texas Public School.

EQUIPMENT AND SUPPLIES

Generally speaking, the normal and the handicapped can use the same type of equipment. Audible balls and jump ropes are a must for the blind, as are large playground-size balls for the youngest children.[2] The J. A. Preston Corporation (71 Fifth Avenue, New York) is one company that has developed many new and imaginative types of equipment for the handicapped. A catalogue describing their products can be obtained from them at the above-mentioned address. Some useful equipment that can be purchased from this company includes

Walking parallel bars	Training walkers
Corner-style staircases	Folding walkers
Suspension ambulators	Full body-suspension walkers
Elgin testing, evaluation, and isometric exercise units	Preston bicycle exercisers
Dumbbell wagons	Tumbling mats
Treadmills with height-adjustable handrails	Stall bars and benches
	Hand exercisers
Scoopball and "safe-t-bat" game kits	Wheelchair training stools
	Rubber horseshoe sets
Folding tennis tables	Table tennis sets
Gym scooter boards	Rug looms
Standing boxes and tables	Electric kilns
Playing card holders and shufflers	Stanley tool sets
Curb blocks and ramps	Utility work tables

---

[2] Beep balls (audio wired for sound) are now available for blind children. They are manufactured by the Denver Council of Telephone Pioneers. For information write Kentucky School for the Blind, Louisville, Kentucky 40205.

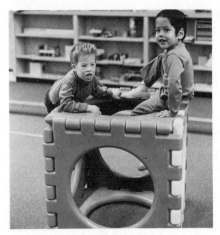 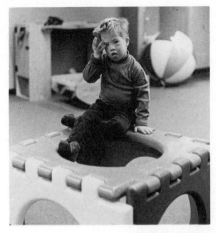

It takes coordinated movements and determination to climb on top of a walk-through block. It can be used to help children develop courage as well as to learn how to climb. Courtesy of the Richardson, Texas Public Schools.

The kinds and amount of equipment and supplies needed depends upon the number, sex, and degree of handicapping defects of those who are to be served in the program as well as available free supplies, skill level of groups, geographical location, and other factors. For games and sports, one basketball or softball bat for every eight students is adequate. Equipment and supplies needed for physical recreation include the following:

Body Building, Physical Fitness, and Figure Control
    Calisthenics—mats
    Body mechanics—mats, full-length mirror
    Weight lifting—weights, bars, collars, head harnesses
    Isometric contractions—head harnesses, straps, hooks on wall, floor, and
       ceiling
    Combative activities—mats
    Relays—stop watch

Individual Sports
    Archery—bows, arrows, arm guards, finger tabs, ground quivers, targets
    Badminton—birds, nets, standards, racquets
    Bowling—bowling balls, pins, alley or plastic balls, and pins with back
       stop
    Golf—balls, iron and wood clubs, driving range or cage
    Tennis—balls, nets, standards, racquets, backstop
    Wrestling—mats, head gear
    Croquet—balls, mallets, wickets
    Deck tennis—rings, nets, standards
    Handball—official handballs and gloves or soft handballs
    Horseshoes—horseshoes, stakes, pits
    Shuffleboard—cues, disks

Track and Field
    Track events—batons, hurdles, stop watch, starting blocks

Field events—tape measure, jumping pits, jumping and vaulting standards, shot put, vaulting poles, javelin, discus

Aquatics

Swimming and diving—flutter boards, diving boards, life-saving equipment, hair dryers

Water polo—balls, goals, hair dryers

Team Sports

Basketball—balls, goals, backboards

Field hockey—balls, goals, sticks, shin pads, goalie pads

Football (tackle, touch, flag)—balls, goalposts, protective equipment, flags

Soccer—balls, goals, protective equipment

Softball and baseball—balls, bats, bases, gloves, protective equipment, backstop

Speedball—balls, football goalposts

Volleyball—balls, nets, standards

Dance

Folk, square, social, modern—piano, records, record player, percussion instruments, full-length mirror

Tumbling and Gymnastics

Tumbling and rebound tumbling—mats, tumbling belt, trampoline

Gymnastics—horizontal bar, ladders, rings, side horse, parallel bars, ropes, vaulting buck, Swedish box, springboard, balance beam

Supplies are also needed for record keeping, the arts and crafts program, table games, social recreation, and dramatics (costumes, makeup supplies, etc.).

It is necessary to make an inventory of supplies and equipment yearly. Such a record will enable the leader to gain helpful information for future program needs as well as to develop budget requests.

Creative leaders soon learn to improvise and use things in their environment for their program. The following items can be made from scrap or inexpensive materials:

Archery—finger tabs from tire inner tubes; arm guards from heavy cardboard and rubber bands; quivers from mailing tubes

Baseball—homeplate, a pitcher's box, backstops from scrap lumber and heavy wire; batting tees made with a heavy wooden base and a hard rubber tube; bases from flattened heavy fire hose held together in base form by nuts and bolts and covered with a heavy material

Basketball—goals from heavy metal rings and heavy string nets

Dance—music for accompaniment from barrel kegs covered with leather, shakers from rock-filled cans; tambourines from tin plates and metal bottle tops; wind and string instruments from scrap materials

Football—goalposts from scrap lumber

Golf—a miniature course, with tin cans driven into the ground for holes and the game played with hockey or broomsticks with varied sizes of balls

Gymnastics—a balance beam and Swedish box from scrap lumber; broomsticks for the stick stunts and balancing; chinning bar, ladder walk, and hanging ropes and ladders from ropes of varying sizes

Recreational activities—box hockey, dart boards and darts, ring toss equipment, tilting spears, tire quoits, toss boards and rings, checkerboards and disks from scrap materials

Shuffleboard—cue sticks and disks from scrap lumber

Soccer, hockey, speedball—goalposts from scrap lumber and heavy chicken wire

Swimming—buoys from rope and wood

Tennis, badminton, volleyball—net posts of wood or iron pipes driven into the ground; a rope for a net; tennis backboards from scrap lumber

Track—starting blocks, jump standards, broad jump take-off board, indicators of broad and high jumps, pole vault standard, shot-put toe circle and toe board from materials available from local lumber companies at little or no cost

Tumbling—mats from bed mattresses that have been discarded or secured from army surplus stores

TRANSPORTATION

Many recreation departments and special schools provide transportation for handicapped persons taking part in their programs. The provision for this should be a vital part of program planning whether the type of transportation be via bus, taxi, or private car. Many departments prefer having their own buses which have built-in safety features such as seats with belts or areas inside to which wheelchairs can be fastened securely to the floor.

Drivers for the handicapped should be carefully selected not only for their ability to drive safely but also for their cheerfulness and attitudes toward both life in general and the handicapped. All bus drivers must have chauffeur licenses. Compact small buses are usually superior to larger ones. Volunteer drivers from service organizations within the community such as the American Red Cross Motor Corps often will provide needed transportation for those not requiring lifting or special handling.

Insurance coverage for all who transport the handicapped is a must from the standpoint of being protected from suits in case of negligence or accidents. However, all drivers should be aware that they are subject to legal suit if negligence on their part can be proven. Those teaching physical activities are especially vulnerable for cases of proven negligence, for accidents sometimes do occur in spite of careful steps taken to prevent them. These leaders can be held liable for proven negligence for any of the following reasons:

1. Pupil injuries as a result of defective playground or gymnastic equipment (Physical educators should check and periodically report in *written form* to their administrators known defective, dangerous equipment and hazardous areas. They should keep a carbon copy of this report.)

2. Injuries that occur to pupils who attempt to do exercises or activities

beyond their skill, such as handstands, running-jump somersaults, etc. (Teachers should not permit students to attempt exercises or activities for which they have not developed the necessary skills or been warned about inherent dangers.)

3. Injuries caused by the negligence of another pupil (The other pupil's misconduct must be foreseeable. All teachers should know about what to expect of each student in behavior as well as performance.)

4. Injuries that occur as a result of inattention to *all* students' activities, *all* the time (Physical educators who teach class by throwing in the ball and leaving, or other such types of instructing by remote control, are *asking for trouble.*)

Leaders of rugged physical activities can safeguard themselves from liability as well as prevent injury to participants if they check all equipment periodically and report any deficiencies, in writing, to supervisors. They must be especially on the lookout for defective playground and other kinds of apparatus, such as worn-out equipment and unattached lockers or other items that could injure students. Leaders must also be sure that all students in the required programs and athletes have had recent physical examinations. All parents must sign yearly permission play forms. Injured students or players should not be sent back into a class or game without clearing with the school physician or other medical personnel. Overly and easily fatigued students or players must be removed from too-strenuous class activity or game play. Students need individual help to develop physical stamina and strength. Students should never be allowed to try a stunt or other physical activity until the necessary lead-up skills have been learned. All students must have mastered the needed skills and game techniques before they are allowed to play in games. Finally, all games should be played according to their rules, with the required number of players on each team. Avoid matching an unskilled player with a highly skilled one in events in which chances of injury are greatly increased (e.g., wrestling and pole vaulting).

SUGGESTED READINGS

Athletic Institute, *Planning Areas and Facilities for Health, Physical Education, and Recreation.* Chicago: The Athletic Institute, Merchandise Mart, 1972.

Challenge (periodic newsletter). Washington, D.C.: American Alliance for Health, Physical Education and Recreation.

Information Center, *Recreation for the Handicapped.* Carbondale, Ill.: Little Grassy Facilities, Southern Illinois University, 1972.

Institute of Rehabilitation Medicine, *The Design of a Pre-School Therapeutic Playground.* New York: New York University Medical Center, 1972.

LUCAS, CAROL, *Recreation in Gerontology.* Springfield, Ill.: Charles Thomas, 1964.

National Therapeutic Recreation Society, *Therapeutic Recreation Annual,* Vol. 7. Arlington, Va., 1970.

PCMR Message. Washington, D.C.: The President's Committee on Mental Retardation, 1971.

Program for the Mentally Retarded (periodical). Washington, D.C.: American Association for Health, Physical Education and Recreation, 1968.

Recreation for the Retarded (periodical). Write the National Association for Retarded Children, 420 Lexington Avenue, New York 10017.

SCHOENBOHM, W. B., *Planning and Operating Facilities for Crippled Children.* Springfield, Ill.: Charles Thomas, 1962.

STEIN, JULIAN, *Special Olympics Instructional Manual* (periodical). Washington, D.C.: American Alliance for Health, Physical Education and Recreation, 1972.

WALTER, FELIX, *Sports Centers and Swimming Pools: A Study of their Design with Reference to the Needs of the Physically Disabled* (periodical). London, England: The Thistle, 1971 (available from the Disabled Living Foundation).

11

The Leader's Role
and Teaching Methods

Special education and adaptive physical education have become recognized educational disciplines with their own body of specialized knowledge and professional preparation requirements. Anyone qualifying as a professional in these fields must

1. Have a broad liberal education background with completed courses in the specific areas of particular specialization
2. Be able to accept responsibility for the consequences of professional actions and judgments
3. Have integrity and be dedicated to the ideal of helping others learn to help themselves
4. Abide by the code of ethics and standards set by this profession
5. Be willing to seek new knowledges and skills in order to increase effectiveness as a professional
6. See the exceptional child or adult as one who is both educationally and recreationally handicapped

This specialist has great responsibility for helping the exceptional reach their highest potential as citizens and human beings able to cope successfully with a variety of life's problems. The properly *educated* handicapped person is a liberated, unique individual who can move about in and explore the environment, respond to and cope with stumbling blocks to progress, and is willing to learn to be both an individual and a contributing group member. The leader's responsibilities center around helping such people learn many new skills for personal development and enjoyment. The skillful leader will be able to make what is to be learned interesting, challenging, and fun.

Special education as such should provide many kinds of multisensory experiences which will be enriching and developmental for each person. These experiences will not only be of diagnostic value—they will also speed up learning and physical improvement. In addition, such experiences will have a preventive function, emphasizing the deletion of failure. Many will be experimental in nature. They will prepare the handicapped person for independent living as well as vocational placement. Highly individualized and continuous, special educational experiences can enable the exceptional person to be a functioning and contributing citizen.

Thus the leader's role is a multiple one—part nursemaid, part judge, part foster parent, part friend and policeman, part teacher and counselor, part learner and specialized experimental expert. The effective leader will be a scholarly practitioner who must constantly explore, improvise, and continually evaluate his or her attempts to find the best ways to help each exceptional person learn how to help himself best according to educationally sound principles and teaching methods. Such a person will realize that a "blueprint designated as universally applicable for all children with a common diagnostic label" [1] is unwise and unproductive.

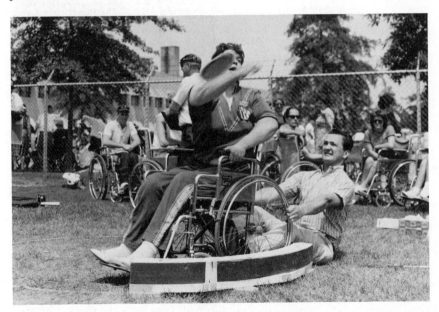

The physical educator does many things besides teaching skills. Courtesy of the National Wheelchair Association.

[1] See Francis Connor, "The Sword and the Spirit," *Exceptional Children* (May 1964), p. 10.

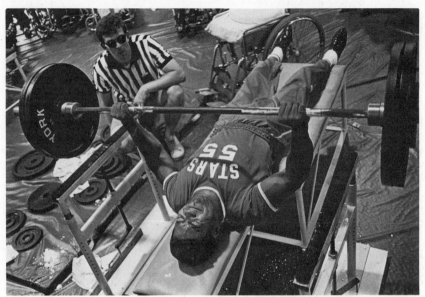

The physical educator should also know how to officiate at competitive events. Courtesy of the AAHPER.

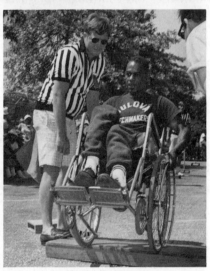

Our society expects teachers to be good models for others, realistic idealists, and good citizens who contribute to the building of a better community, nation, and future. The special educator must have in addition a good sense of humor, skill in working with parents as well as their atypical offspring, and a knowledge of community agencies and national associations from which help can be obtained when needed. It is imperative that this person be a team member working with others in institutions, hospitals, private homes, the school, and the community to provide the richest possible kind of educational experiences for each exceptional child and adult.

Learning can be a thrilling adventure or drudgery. It is in the teacher's power to make it a positive, challenging, and satisfying life

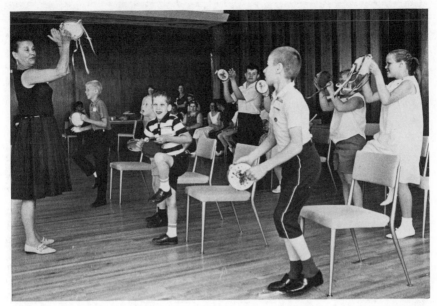

The success of any educational program is based in part upon good administrators, but it is based most of all upon the skill, warmth, enthusiasm, and the love of teachers. Courtesy of the AAHPER.

experience. Learning takes place wherever there is life. Students learn best under the guidance of teachers who help them develop desirable behavior patterns, a workable philosophy of life, and a sense of values in harmony with our societal ideals.

All human learning evolves around these six basic categories:

1. Motor skills
2. Meanings, concepts, and generalizations
3. Attitudes, interests, and motives
4. Social and emotional control
5. Esthetic appreciation
6. Problem solving

What we learn comes to us through our five senses. The more these senses are combined within the learning experience, the greater and more lasting learning will be. What we see *and* hear is a richer educational experience for us than what we merely hear *or* see. Learning means mastery over experience, resulting in changed behavior. If we do not profit from our experiences, we have not learned. We learn when we

1. Understand words or symbols and their meaning
2. Can communicate with others
3. Develop and use new skills
4. Form new habits
5. Develop new interests
6. Gain new understandings and insights
7. Make generalizations from learned facts

167

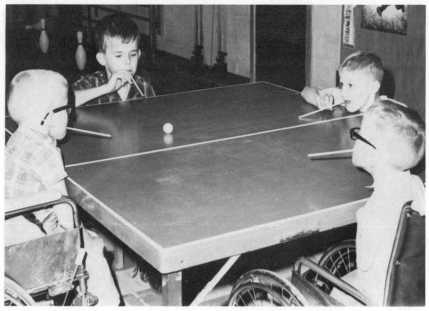

These children are learning much about each other while playing this game. Courtesy of the AAHPER.

8. Develop and refine social skills
9. Become concerned about our environment and others around us, and develop ethical values which govern our behavior
10. Develop a realistic self-image
11. Show concern for the rights of others
12. Have respect for and obey laws

The most frequently found types of learning are (1) *conditioned responses* (the formation of patterned reflex actions); (2) *autogenous* (self-initiated) *responses;* (3) *sociogenous responses* (the result of social stimulation); (4) *incidental learning* (the result of exposure to stimuli—for

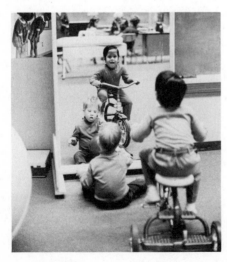

Gaining a good self image is basic to learning. Courtesy of the Richardson, Texas Public Schools.

example, learning to ride a bicycle more safely after seeing an accident caused by carelessness); and (5) *insightful learning* (the result of suddenly seeing the relationship of several parts with a learning process).

Education is a long, slow process that is fostered by the school, the home, and the community. Much of any student's attitude toward his own ability to learn is a reflection of how others have regarded or labeled him—his family, peers, and those at school and in the community.

LEARNING PRINCIPLES

Basic teaching beliefs and action guides are principles resulting from experience, research, and education. The best learning will result if the following learning principles are used as action springboards:

1. *The learner teaches himself.* It is only by one's own trial-error attempts that a person learns. An important function of the teacher is to provide motivation, guiding the student in his or her attempts, and helping in the evaluation of these attempts.

2. *All learning results from trying.* Discovery can only come from searching. We learn from doing, not from being told or watching others perform. One must try for himself and through his own unique experience gain skill, understanding, knowledge, and appreciation.

3. *The learner controls the learning situation and what he will learn.* If the student feels secure and confident, the rate of progress increases. It is detrimental to be without any autonomy in what, when, and how to learn. Knowledge of personal progress in relationship to that of others can be an asset or a liability, depending upon the amount of self-confidence and emotional drive the person has, and the potency of the desire to learn. Much of the drive and will to learn comes from being allowed to control what and how much one learns.

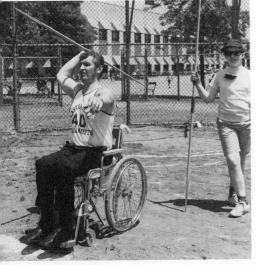

The learner teaches himself. Courtesy of the National Wheelchair Athletic Association.

4. *Each person learns in his own way.* Learning is a unique experience and each person goes about it differently. Each also develops an individual learning curve. For most, this curve will rise quickly at first, taper off to a plateau, then rise again as the learner becomes more aware that victory is in sight.

5. *Overlearning leads to longer retention.* Practice does *not* make perfect unless one is practicing perfectly. However, practice makes *permanent.* It is harder to unlearn than to learn correctly.

6. *Emotions retard or accelerate learning.* Fear and insecurity block learning and dam up desire to learn; confidence and encouragement foster learning. (These facts are especially pertinent in teaching the handicapped.)

7. *Short practice periods are superior to long ones.* The pupil's attention span is the key here. A learning pause can bring real refreshment, as well as desired results, more quickly.

8. *Transfer will occur when situations are recognized to be alike.* Transferring of learning takes place only when the learner actually perceives similarities. The child who can see and feel the relationship of the baseball throw to the tennis serve will learn the latter more quickly if he can throw a baseball well.

9. *Learning can be an exciting, challenging adventure.* People, and especially children, are eager to try new things, to learn to master them and be challenged by them.

10. *Evaluation is an essential part of learning.* To learn best, one must have the learning task or goal well in mind. To profit most from any attempts to learn, it is necessary to know where errors were made and why.

TEACHING METHODS

Just as adequate professional preparation is necessary for successful teaching, so also is the careful planning of each lesson. This can best be done by the whole-part-whole method, for which the teacher begins by (1) planning the course content for a semester or a single unit, (2) devising plans for each class period of this larger whole, and (3) evaluating the results at the unit's completion.

Group plans are the prerequisites for successful group experiences. Consequently, the teacher and pupils should together set up desired individual goals and class objectives, choose the materials to be mastered, share a teaching-learning experience, and then measure their success or failure to obtain goals.

Many teaching methods are valuable, but there are times when one is superior to another. The one best to use depends upon ever-changing factors which the successful instructor learns to sense or feel. Any method is only worthy of use if through it, desired results can be obtained and it is socially approved. A teaching method that has proven to be successful for one teacher may be a failure for another. Ways of teaching others are patterns that must be tailored to fit individual situations. Some of the many techniques for successful teaching of the handicapped include

Chalk talks	Experiments
Drills	Class discussions
Lectures	Workshops
Questions and answers	Forums
Reports	Assignments
Demonstrations and participation	Field trips
	Debates
Supervised practice	Workbooks
Role playing	Projects
Visual aids	Combinations of all listed

Teaching Motor Skills

Movement accuracy results from practicing correct movement patterns until they become habitual. Because it is harder to unlearn or break a faulty movement habit in order to relearn or replace it with an accurate one than it is to learn the correct movement initially, it is best for a beginner learning any sport to practice under skilled guidance. Some factors that contribute to the correct performance of any movement skill are [2]

1. Strength
2. Energy
3. Ability to change directions
4. Body flexibility
5. Agility
6. Peripheral vision
7. Good vision
8. Concentration
9. An understanding of the mechanics of the movement
10. An absence of disturbing emotional complications

One's own personal drives, needs, and abilities determine how fast skills are learned, as do one's degree of innate coordination and type of body build. Factors that speed up skill learning are the presence of spectators, the size of the group, the degree of group interaction, the kinds of and amount of pressure applied by the teacher upon the learner, and the competition between individuals or groups. Because each individual reacts to these factors in a different way, the teacher must be willing to experiment in order to discover the best way to spark each person's learning. Anxiety, stress, tension, fatigue, and repeated failure are learn-

---

[2] Bryant Cratty, *Movement Behavior and Motor Learning* (Philadelphia: Lea & Febiger, 1964), p. 43.

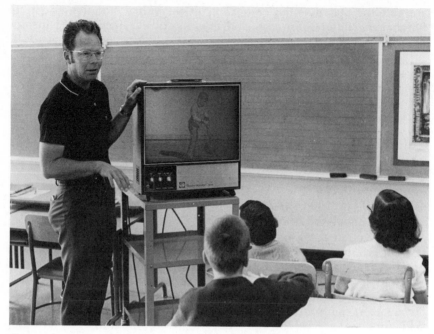

Game rules can be learned in a variety of ways. Courtesy of the Los Angeles Public Schools.

ing checkreins. Age and maturation level determine what skills can best be learned at a given time. For most elementary school children, activities that evolve around big-muscle movements such as are found in running or jumping are quickly and eagerly learned. Intricate movements that require coordination of the small muscles of the body are more difficult and less appropriate for younger children. Students who learn skills rapidly are usually more highly motivated and above average in strength and intelligence and can analyze quickly the correct body mechanics needed in order to perform more refined movements correctly. Because there are only a few students of this caliber in any class, unless it is homogeneously grouped, teachers often call upon these most highly skilled individuals for demonstration purposes or as teaching assistants. This practice should only be followed, however, if such students are also given opportunities to polish more brilliantly their own physical, social, mental, and leadership skills. And it should not be used at the expense of the confidence of other students.

Although students can learn skills without a teacher, the most rapid and efficient skill learning results from copying, guidance, correction, and skillful instructor suggestion. All learning comes from trial, error, and insight, in that order. Mistakes are basic to mastery, for without them there cannot be learning.

Immediate evaluation and correction is vital to learning speed and accuracy. Verbal instructions in the first phase of learning should be kept

Safety	—Always be safety-conscious and remember that accidents are the chief cause of death among children.
Try	—Try always to make your program better and yourself a better leader/teacher.
Utilization	—Make the best possible use of your community resources, your abilities, and your intelligence.
Variety	—Add variety to your program and keep it up to date. Be creative and draw upon the creativity of the participants for new program highlights.
Work	—Work your hardest to be a better teacher.
"Xamine"	—Continually examine your teaching methods and make sure you are up-to-date in your knowledge of the handicapped.
You	—Remember that you as a leader must look and act like a leader. You have it in *your* power to contribute in a major way to the success, happiness, and well-being of other human beings.
Zest	—Remember that enthusiasm is as contagious as measles. Be zestful!

SUGGESTED READINGS

CLARKE, H. H., and D. H. CLARKE, *Developmental and Adapted Physical Education*. Englewood Cliffs, N.J.: Prentice-Hall, 1963.

HAMMERMAN, DONALD, and W. M. HAMMERMAN, *Teaching in the Outdoors*. Minneapolis: Burgess, 1964.

LAWTHER, JOHN, *The Learning of Physical Skills*. Englewood Cliffs, N.J.: Prentice-Hall, 1968.

National Easter Seal Society for Crippled Children and Adults, "Educational Therapy," *Rehabilitation Literature*, 31, No. 4 (April 1970).

————, "The Disadvantaged and Counseling," *Rehabilitation Literature*, 31, No. 7 (July 1970).

OXENDINE, JOSEPH, *Psychology of Motor Learning*. New York: Appleton-Century, 1968.

VANNIER, MARYHELEN, and HALLY BETH POINDEXTER, *Individual and Team Sports for Girls and Women*. Philadelphia: W. B. Saunders, 1976.

VANNIER, MARYHELEN, and HOLLIS FAIT, *Teaching Physical Education in Secondary Schools*, 4th ed. Philadelphia: W. B. Saunders, 1975.

12

Program Activities

A physical activities program for the handicapped may be corrective, modified, or developmental. Or it can be all three, depending upon activities selected for the curriculum, the degree of handicap of persons taking part in the program, and the skill of the teacher.

The total physical activities program should consist of the core instructional program and the elective sports program (intramurals, extramurals, and interscholastic competition). This program should be closely related to school programs in health education, recreation, and outdoor education.

The activities program for children as well as older youth must be built upon sound educational principles. These stress that the program should be

1. Based upon the age, sex, needs, capabilities, and interests of the students
2. Related to the physical, mental, social, and emotional characteristics of each individual and group
3. Planned in light of the objectives, aims, and goals sought by the teacher and class
4. Established to make the best use of all available resources, including teacher qualifications and facilities and equipment available at the school and in the community
5. Wide enough in scope to be of present and future value to each individual, as well as the community, state, and nation
6. One that can be participated in safely and that will lead to an improved state of health

7. Rich in opportunities to develop desirable behavior patterns
8. A learning laboratory for democratic group living
9. Flexible, with provision for student choice of activities
10. Coeducational in part
11. Planned to foster all degrees of skill—beginning, intermediate, and advanced

If at all possible, the handicapped child and adult should be taught physical activities in a class with the normal. This, of course, depends upon the degree of handicapping conditions each has. Some need instruction on a one-to-one basis whereas others can be taught in small groups either in homogeneous or heterogeneous groups.

Classification of Activities

Activities in the program should include (1) the fundamental movement skills incorporated into games and individual and team sports; (2) formal activities and gymnastics; (3) aquatics; (4) self-testing activities; (5) dance; and (6) recreational activities including hiking and camping.

Class Management

The well-organized, specialized professional physical educator should conduct classes in the most efficient manner possible. In addition, care should be taken that a positive attitude is maintained by attention to such details as the leader's manner (including clean, neat uniform as well as a good teaching attitude) and what goes on before and after classes. The students' attitude toward the class is affected by what goes on in the shower room or locker room as well as the playing field, gym, or pool.

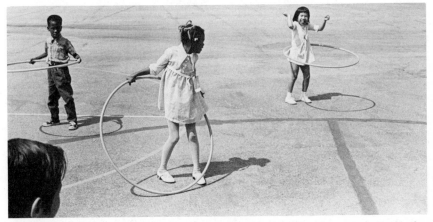

Self-testing activities should be a vital part of the physical education program for children. Courtesy of the Los Angeles Public Schools.

Carefully planned, routinized class procedures save both time and energy. Superior teachers are those who make the best use of each precious class hour to obtain desired results according to standards devised by professional association and leading experts in their field.

Effective teaching results in meaningful student learning. If physical activities are taught to help students gain a secure place in the world, those in charge of educational and rehabilitation programs for the handicapped must be sure that the quality of these programs is excellent. Careful planning and good organization are basic to effective teaching of every class, every day.

Because instructional periods are short, the teacher must find shortcuts in order to be able to devote the major part of every class period to teaching. Conditioning students to respond quickly and automatically to habits of undressing and dressing, roll-call procedures, checking equipment in and out, and many other automatic movement patterns, saves many minutes in each class hour. The teacher, likewise, should be conditioned to efficiently perform the numerous marginal tasks necessary in conducting such classes.

ROLL-TAKING

Roll-taking should be done quickly and accurately. Here are some suggested methods for doing so:

1. By squads—the squad leader is responsible for finding out who is absent from his squad.

    Advantage: Allows for leadership training. Roll is taken quickly.
    Disadvantage: Could allow for cheating. The teacher does not learn the students' names and faces so quickly.

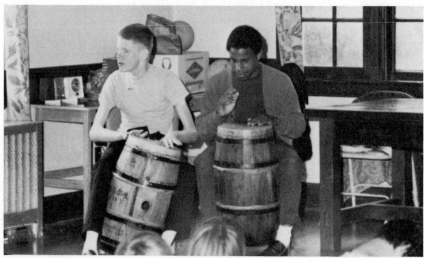

Students should be encouraged to practice skills after class. Courtesy of the California School for the Blind.

2. By seating plan—the teacher marks down names or numbers of vacant seating or standing places.

> *Advantage:*   Fairly quick method for taking role. The teacher is better able to coordinate names with faces.
>
> *Disadvantage:* Does not allow for leadership training. Takes more time than squad method.

3. Roll-call—the teacher calls the roll with students answering if present.

> *Advantage:*   Teacher may learn students' names with very little effort. Teacher may be assured about who is present or absent.
>
> *Disadvantage:* Too time-consuming. Allows for no leadership training.

Each teacher should develop his or her own system for recording absences, tardinesses, and excuses from daily participation. Roll should be taken at the beginning of each class period. Requiring each pupil to wear a name tag will enable the teacher to learn each child's name more quickly; this, in turn, is a means of class control.

Individual record cards should be filled out the first day the class meets and permanent record cards kept on each student. Here grades, intramural points earned, physical fitness test scores, teacher's comments and other information should be recorded.

CLOTHING

Recommended clothing for boys are dark trunks, cotton tee-shirts high-top tennis shoes, and wool socks. Girls may wear shorts and blouses, low-cut tennis shoes, and wool socks. One-piece uniforms are favored by some teachers. Regulation clothing for both groups may be required or each class member may be given the opportunity to wear what he wishes. These clothing may be purchased locally or through manufacturers, most of whom advertise regularly in the *Journal of Health, Physical Education and Recreation.* Each agency should devise a plan whereby students financially unable to buy shorts and tops may be assisted in obtaining them. Students should be encouraged to wear clean clothing. Since wearing street clothes inhibits freedom of movement, every person in the class should be asked to wear apparel which is comfortable, stretchable, and durable.

Students should be provided with clean towels or be required to bring their own. They should be encouraged to take a shower after taking part in vigorous activities.

CLASS ORGANIZATION

Physical activity classes should be kept small. Lack of sufficient time, poor facilities and inadequate equipment, and large numbers of pupils or several with severe handicaps present many problems to the teacher. Careful planning for the best type of class organization possible will yield more fruitful results. Students, as well as volunteers in the community, should assist the instructor in planning, conducting, and evaluating the program on each grade level, when possible.

Skillful organization and wise planning will assure that each period of instruction is both meaningful to the learners and educationally sound. The program itself should be kept flexible and provide individuals taking part in it to enjoy what they are doing as well as to have freedom of choice and action. The classes should be conducted informally but should always be well-controlled.

The teacher should have a definite beginning and ending to each class period. The students must be conditioned to listen automatically when the leader is talking, to form into a circle or squad formation when the class starting signal is given, and to sit in assigned groups at the end of each class for a short evaluative discussion of the period. Because students experiment with each new leader in order to learn how far they can go or how much they can get away with, it is of primary importance that beginning with the first class, the teacher be *firm, fair,* and *consistent* in methods used for controlling the group. Good class organization helps all students feel secure and ready for each new challenging experience, and this is especially true of the handicapped.

FORMATION FOR INSTRUCTION

Far too much precious class time can be lost by reorganizing groups for relays, teams, or skill drills. In order to eliminate such waste, students should be conditioned to form quickly into desired groups when directed. Squads or teams of six to ten in number usually are best. Placing each group to cover the floor area fully allows the teacher to supervise the entire class effectively. The following formations can be learned and formed quickly. (In each, SL means student leader.)

Fan

Players are spread before the leader in a fan formation (Figure 12–1). This is especially effective in skill drills for throwing, catching, and kicking balls of various sizes. The teacher works as a group supervisor.

Line

This is the easiest of all formations (Figure 12–2) for beginners to learn. It is good for relays, basket shooting, and games in which children take turns. Not more than five should be in each line, if possible.

Circle

Groups can get into a circle (Figure 12–3) quickly from the line or fan formation by following their leader. This formation is especially good for simple games and ball skill drills with the leader in the center throwing the ball to each player and correcting faulty movements when it is thrown back.

Shuttle

This grouping (Figure 12–4) is best for ball passing or kicking skill drills.

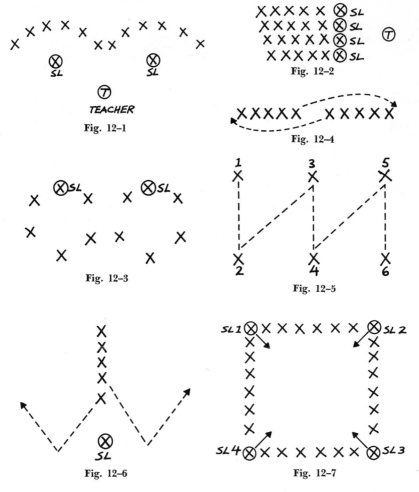

Fig. 12-1

Fig. 12-2

Fig. 12-4

Fig. 12-3

Fig. 12-5

Fig. 12-6

Fig. 12-7

Zigzag

Two lines face each other. Player 1 throws to 2 who throws to 3, etc. This formation is best for soccer kicking, volleying, throwing, and catching.

Corner

The leader facing the line gives signal for 1 and 2 to form a V corner (Figure 12–6). The odd numbers go right; the even to the left. This grouping is ideal for skill drills and teaching response to command movements necessary for marching.

Square

Have four groups form a square (Figure 12–7). Squad 1 forms west; 2 north; 3 east; 4 south. The leader stands to the left of his squad. This one is effective for ball-passing drills and team games such as line dodgeball.

181

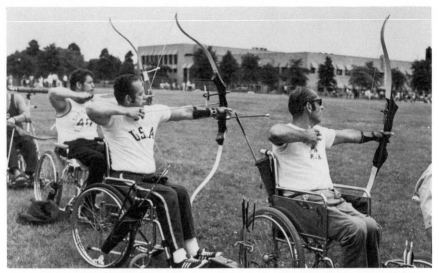

Homogeneous grouping is often best for teaching new skills. Courtesy of the AAHPER.

METHODS OF GROUPING

A wide variety of student groups should be used throughout the year. Providing opportunities for many students to be squad leaders and team captains is advisable. Suggested means of grouping pupils include those determined by

1. Class or age
2. The skilled (as determined by skill tests or observation)
3. Numbering off by 2's, 3's, or 4's, depending upon class size
4. Electing captains and having each one choose his team (Although this may be used infrequently, care must be taken that those chosen last become group leaders or gain recognition in other activities.)
5. Dividing the tallest members among various squads
6. Teacher-formed teams or squads
7. Special skill practice groups
8. Dividing a circle in half
9. Asking three in the class to stand in front of you and then direct the rest to line up behind any one of these persons (This is the quickest way to form teams.)
10. Dividing the class by numbers (e.g., the first ten go to one corner to tumble, the next ten go to another corner to do relays, etc.)
11. Dividing same as above, except pupils are allowed to choose the activity and equipment they wish
12. Physical size

Throughout the year, the teacher should stress the qualities of democratic leadership and the duties and responsibilities of a good team captain or squad leader.

USE OF STUDENT LEADERS

A good leader often leads from behind. If an important element of teaching is guiding people to learn how to become independent and

182

grow as individuals, then boys and girls must learn early in life how to solve their own and group problems, how to cooperate, choose leaders, and follow as well as lead others.

The use of a student leader can produce more efficient, effective teaching. It can also enable the teacher to work more in the role of a supervisor. As soon as possible, the pupils should select the leaders they believe to be most qualified. A Leader's Club may be organized among teenagers as a means of teaching students how to lead. This group should meet regularly with the teacher to plan activities, develop physical skills, evaluate the work to be done with the rest of the group, and learn new activities to be presented later in class. Student leaders may serve for four months or be changed more frequently. The former method adds unity to the program as well as increasing leadership skills; the latter method passes leadership opportunities around.

THE LEADER'S CONDUCT

Leaders who are alert, poised, calm, assured, enthusiastic, and controlled can evoke the confidence of other class members. Traits necessary for good class leadership are appearance, cleanliness, dependability, forcefulness, promptness, instructional skill, and good group control.

Before class the teacher should be dressed in a costume that allows freedom of movement. If possible, each pupil should be greeted by name as he or she enters the play area. (Requiring students to wear name tags will help here.) All needed equipment for the class should be ready and the activities to be taught should be well planned.

CHECKING EQUIPMENT IN AND OUT

If there is no custodian available for checking equipment, procedures for doing so should be established. Assigning one student in each group to this responsibility is recommended. All equipment needed for each period should be carefully checked as a safety precaution, and all items should be readily accessible so that they can be gathered at one time. Large strong laundry sacks are ideal for this purpose and are easily carried back and forth to playing fields.

MOVING TO OTHER AREAS

Groups should be moved quickly from indoor to outdoor play areas. Methods for speeding up the laggers are to require all to run to and from the assigned areas, and to vitalize teaching of the activity so that students are eager for class to begin. The physical activity instructional program should be like a merry-go-round. If it is enjoyable, adventurous, and satisfying enough, youth will want to jump on and keep going with the group.

SHOWERS AND LOCKER ROOMS

Each student should know where to put his clothing when changing for class. Each should lock his locker before coming into the gym.

A combination lock is recommended and the leader should have a master key.

Students should be encouraged, but not required, to take showers and be given enough time for showering and dressing after the class. Some few will find their greatest joy in this part of the program, especially those from low-income groups who do not have adequate bathing facilities at home.

The shower and locker rooms should be supervised, preferably at all times, by a custodian. If this is impossible, it is necessary that the leader do so as each group enters, showers, and leaves. Horseplay should be forbidden as a safety precaution. Rules regarding smoking, marking on walls or using obscene language must be obeyed throughout the entire building, and especially here during the free play and/or recreational period. The leader should assume the authority necessary to protect public and private property. Experienced leaders realize that often they do their best teaching outside the activity class while talking informally to individuals in the locker room or on the way to and from the playing field.

KEEPING RECORDS

Records should be functional and practical, and used as a means of evaluating student progress and program content, or for recording administrative details. They should not be time-consuming or energy-draining for the leader. Such records include essential health information, basket or locker master sheets, cumulative physical activity parental permit forms, attendance records, inventory and accident reports. Records and grade reports should be kept in a locked steel file. All recorded information should be for present or future use, for accurate and meaningful reports are as essential to good teaching as efficient and effective class management.

PROGRAM FOR ELEMENTARY-AGE CHILDREN

The total program for both the lower and upper elementary grades should be a balanced one and contain a wide range of activities. Broad areas around which the program should be built are:

1. Rhythmic activities
2. Games of low organization
3. Relays
4. Movement exploration
5. Camping and outdoor education (grades 4, 5, 6)
6. Lead-up athletic team games
7. Aquatics
8. Stunts and self-testing activities
9. Posture and the fundamental skills of human movement

Planning the Program

Points to consider when building the daily, weekly, monthly, or a longer program in physical activities include (1) the age group, (2) the number in the class, (3) sex, (4) interest and needs of the pupils, (5) the carryover value of the activities, and (6) the available facilities and equipment.

The leader should form both general and specific objectives for the class to accomplish. General objectives may be to increase physical fitness, skill range and accuracy, knowledge, improve attitudes and appreciation, and make better use of leisure time. Specific objectives the leader wishes to accomplish with the group may include developing in each child

1. Good health, happiness, character, and a democratic spirit
2. Leadership and "followership" skills
3. Basic skills in as many kinds of activities as possible
4. Abilities to plan, conduct, and evaluate the learning experience
5. Good safety habits
6. Proper attitudes toward playing, winning, losing; also toward oneself and others
7. Ability to reason and to give directions
8. Independence
9. Integration of health and safety education with physical activity
10. Courage and initiative
11. Vigor and physical fitness
12. Skills in games and activities suitable for after-school play

PERIOD DIVISIONS

Children of elementary age should have a total of one hour daily devoted to physical activity instruction. For those younger, at least 30 minutes daily should be given to class instruction and the remainder of the time to supervised play on the playground. It is customary to have the morning time given over to the former, and the afternoon to supervised free play. Grades 4 to 6 should also have one hour daily for physical education. The suggested time division is 40 minutes for class instruction, with the remaining 20 minutes for supervised playground work later. Some schools devote three 60-minute periods weekly to health instruction. It goes without saying that for the handicapped in this age bracket, physical education is a vital part of school or institutional program. The total amount of time spent on such activities depends largely on the specific disabilities of the children involved.

Regardless of the period divisions, any physical activity period should be carefully planned. Moreover, there should be a spread of activities so that skill mastery can be accomplished.

In the primary grades, emphasis should be placed upon joyful

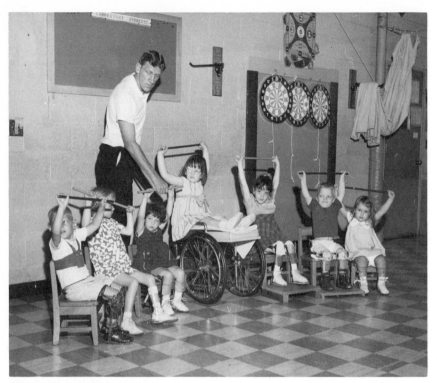

Every day should be a day of learning and a part of each day should be spent having fun. Courtesy of the AAHPER.

activity; small children are not as interested in learning how to do intricate game skills as they are in being active and having fun. On the upper elementary level, however, the teacher should begin to place emphasis on skill, realizing that pupils will receive greater pleasure from games when they can play them with better than average ability.

Instead of including a wide variety of activities in the beginning of the year, the teacher should start with games familiar to the pupils and gradually introduce new ones into the program. She should go from the known to the unknown, reviewing the familiar and gradually including the new.

Pupils and the teacher should evaluate together their weekly and daily progress. Time allotment for this purpose may be 5 minutes daily or 20 to 30 minutes weekly. During this period, the group should plan with the teacher the ensuing work, check progress made toward reaching desired goals and objectives, and discuss problems that have arisen during class time.

Lesson plans for each group should be made weekly, and specific objectives for both the group and each person in it should be kept uppermost in mind. Some activities suitable and recommended for each grade level include:

GRADE 1

Rhythmic Activities

Folk Dance
  I See You
  Shoemaker's Dance
  Danish Dance of Greeting
  Chimes of Dunkirk
  Farmer in the Dell

Singing Games
  A-Hunting We Will Go
  How Do You Do, My Partner?
  London Bridge
  Hokey Pokey
  Muffin Man
  Soldier Boy

Movement Exploration
  Walk to music or rhythm
  Skip to music or rhythm
  Slide to music or rhythm
  Hop to music or rhythm
  Gallop to music or rhythm
  Creative movements to changing
    beats

Games of Low Organization
  Have You Seen My Sheep?
  Crows and Cranes
  Dodgeball
  Fox and Geese
  Flying Dutchman
  Cat and Rat
  Squirrel and Trees
  I Say Stoop
  Slap Jack
  Circle Pass Ball
  Old Mother Witch
  Jump the Brook
  Statues

Stunts, Tumbling, and Self-testing
    Activities
  Log roll
  Forward roll
  Push-up from knees
  Running
  Jumping
  Activities on the jungle gym

GRADE 2

Rhythmic Activities

Folk Dance
  Bleking
  Kinder Polka
  Gustaf's Skoal
  Seven Jumps
  The Crested Hen
  Broom Dance
  Rovenacka

Relay
  Back to back
  Automobile relay
  Head balance relay
  Rope skip relay
  Passing relay
  Stiff-legged relay
  Gunny sack relay
  Three-legged race relay
  Running
  Skipping
  One-leg hop
  Run-up, walk-back
  Running backwards
  Up and over

  Balance relay
  Up and under
  Box relay
  Sack relay

Mimetics and Story Plays
  Rope jumping
  Figure skating
  Branding cows
  Fishing
  Bicycling
  Acting-out sports
  Animals
  Follow the leader
  Building a house
  Trip to the country
  Cowboys and Indians
  Christmas tree and Santa
  Playing in the wind
  Going to the grocery store
  Modes of travel

Singing Games
  Farmer in the Dell
  Hippety Hop to the Barber Shop
  Thread Follows the Needle

I'm Very, Very Tall
The Muffin Man
Old King Cole

Movement Exploration
Combinations of movements
Skip-hop-glide
Changing directions
Changing tempo

*Stunts, Tumbling, and Self-testing
  Activities*
Bear walk
Duck walk
Elephant walk
Seal walk
One-leg hop, changing directions
Log-roll
Rope jumping
Wheelbarrow

Measuring worm
Crab walk
Leap frog
Rocking horse
Chicken fight

Games of Low Organization
Do This–Do That
Midnight
Call Ball
Charley over the Water
Steal the Bacon
Poison Tag
Garden Scamp
Squat Tag
Red Light
Wood Tag
Line Dodgeball

GRADE 3

Rhythmic Activities

Folk Dance
Polka
Ace of Diamonds
Green Sleeves
Indian War Dance
Norwegian Mountain Dance
Tantoli
Finger Polka

Dance Fundamentals
Singing
Gallop
Slides
Fox trot
Polka
Dances created to songs, poems, and
  stories

Movement Exploration
Actions for poems and stories
Song titles
A bus ride
A train trip
The airplane
Gardening
Acting-out sports

Team Games
Soccer Keepaway
Capture the Flag
Kickball
Dodgeball

Boundary Ball
Kick It and Run
Throw It and Run
Line Soccer
Corner Dodgeball

Relays
All four relay
Throw and sit relay
Down and up relay
Soccer dribble relay
Run and throw back relay
Automobile relay
Goal butting
Basketball pass
Horse and rider

Singing Games
Jenny Crack Corn
Captain Jinks
Indian Braves
Looby Lou
Pop Goes the Weasel
Rig-A-Jig
The Needle's Eye

Games of Low Organization
Caboose
Stride Ball
Bull in the Ring
Three Deep
Boiler Burst
New York

Target Throw
Last Couple Out
Hill Dill
Circle Blub Bowls
Line Dodgeball
Hopscotch
Loose Caboose

*Stunts, Tumbling, and Self-testing
    Activities*
Knee dip
Cartwheel

Nip-up
Coffee grinder
Push-up
Cross leg stand
Foot clap
Walrus walk
Backward and forward roll
Chimney
Fish hawk dive
Twister
The swan

GRADE 4

Rhythmic Activities

Folk Dance
Minuet
Broom Dance
Highland Schottische
Seven Jumps
Sellinger's Round
Sailor's Hornpipe
Maine Mixer

Square Dance
Grand March
Virginia Reel
Red River Valley
Take a Little Peek
Jump Jim Crow
Soldier's Joy

Dance, Fundamentals
Walk, run, jump, hop to even rhythm
Skip, slide, gallop, leap to uneven
    rhythm
Creative movements of work, play,
    sports
Creative dance to records
Waltz
Schottische

Games of Low Organization
Hook-on
Streets and Alleys
Vis-à-Vis
Animal Chase
Red Rover
May I?
Charades
Skin the Snake
Merry-Go-Round
Simple Pyramids
Headstand

Nip-up
Cartwheels
Running
Jumping

Team Games
Soccer Dodgeball
Pin Soccer
End Ball
Club Snatch
Bronco Tag
Ankle Tag
Prisoner's Base
Nine-Court Keepaway
Field Ball
Skills of Baseball

Camping and Outing
Hiking
Compass reading
Trail blazing
Fire building
Wood gathering
Menu planning
Outdoor cooking
Garbage disposal
Blanket rolling
Crafts from native materials
Camp project
Fishing

Relays
Rescue relay
Rope-climb relay
Kangaroo relay
Leapfrog relay
Run, throw, catch relay
Goal shooting relay
Zigzag relay
Skip-rope relay

Family relay
Rabbit-jump relay
Soccer relay
Basketball couple passing
Goal shooting
Football pass couple relay
*Stunts, Tumbling, and Self-testing
   Activities*
Chinning
Rope jumping
Goal shooting
Soccer kick for distance
Soccer kick for accuracy
One-leg squat
Jump the stick
Push- and pull-ups
Kickball
Corner kickball
German batball
Newcomb
Captain ball

Base football
Schlagball
Aquatics (Minimum Skills)
Fear elimination
Floating
Crawl
Elementary Gymnastics
Conditioning and free exercises
Balance beam
Stall bars
Stairs
Track and Field
25-yard dash
Standing broad jump
Pull-up and/or jump and reach
Softball throw for distance and
   accuracy
Improvised Events
Field Events

GRADE 5

Rhythmic Activities
Folk Dance
Starlight Schottische
Highland Schottische
Irish Washerwoman
Varsovienne
Kerry Dance
Troika
Sextur
Trip to Helsinki
Sicilian Tarantella
Square Dance
Oh, Johnny
Sally Goodin
Around That Couple, Take a Peek
Chase the Snake
Swing the Girl Behind You
Arkansas
Dance Fundamentals
Fox trot
Waltz hesitation
Skip, slide, gallop
Jump and hop
Space aspects of movement
Striking and dodging
Dance creations
Games of Low Organization
Keep It Up

Pinch-O
Cross Tag
Fire on the Mountain
Wood Tag
Buddy Spud
Keepaway
Relays
Siamese twin relay
Jump-the-stick relay
Human croquet
Rope-jumping relay
Running at increased distances
Squat, jump relay
Juggle relay
Pony express relay
Base-running relay
Aquatics
Crawl
Backstroke
Sidestroke
Elementary diving
Elementary lifesaving
*Stunts, Tumbling, and Self-testing
   Activities*
Russian bear dance
Jump the stick
Hand wrestle
Human bridge

High kick
Dive
Handstand
Seal slap
Jump over stool
Track and field events
Indian leg wrestle
Stick wrestle
Rope skipping for speed and time
Bar hanging by arms, knees
Turn over on low-bar

Camping and Outing
Hiking
Compass reading
Trail blazing
Fire building-reflector, oven, criss-
  cross, travels
Wood chopping
Wood sawing
Menu planning
Outdoor cooking
Garbage disposal
Blanket rolling
Fishing, hunting
Crafts from native materials
Simple shelter construction
Camp soil conservation project
Overnight camping

Team Games
Progressive Dodgeball
Volleyball
Schlagball

Base Football
Softball
Touch Football
Double Dodgeball
Basketball—Twenty-one, Horse
Drop in, Drop out
Circle goal shooting
Basketball pass variations
Soccer
Tennis
Speedball

Track and Field
Obstacle relays
50-yard dash
100-yard dash
440-yard run or fast walk
Broad jump
Low hurdles
Track meet

Elementary Gymnastics
Conditioning and free exercises
Swinging and traveling rings
Side horse
Rope climb
Foot and leg climb
Stirrup climb
Rolled mat activities
Still rings
Elementary flying rings
Rope climbing, single rope
Elementary horizontal bar

GRADE 6

Rhythmic Activities
Folk Dance
Kerry Dance
Sicilian Circle
Irish Song Dance
Jesse Polka
Badger Gavotte
Raatikko
Cherkessia
Road to the Isles
Jarabe Tapatio
Trilby
Laces and Graces
Ranger Polka

Square Dance
Arkansas Traveler
Birdie in the Cage

Heel and Toe Polka
Cotton-Eyed Joe
Rye Waltz
Dive for the Oyster

Dance Fundamentals
Slide
Schottische variations
Waltz
Waltz variations
Congo
Lifting and carrying
Swinging
Propulsive and sustained movements
Dance creations

Games of Low Organization
Stealing Sticks
Ante Over

Horseshoes
Hand Tennis
Box Hockey
Tug-of-War
Broom Hockey
Keepaway
Giant Volleyball
Overtake Softball
Long Base
Target Toss

Relays
Shuttle-pass-soccer relay
Obstacle-dribble relay
Dribble and pass relay
Bounce, pass, and shoot relay
Base-running relays

Stunts and Tumbling
Throwing, batting, kicking for
accuracy
Throwing, batting, kicking for
distance
Base running
Standing broad jump
Hop, step, and jump
Sprinting
The top
Knee-spring
Handstand
Floor dip
Dives
Push- and pull-ups
Pyramids
Simple apparatus

Camping and Outing
Hiking
Bicycle trip camping
Use of two-handed axe
Making things with knife, with
hatchet
Overnight camping utilizing all
skills learned for sleeping,
playing, and cooking in
the woods

Fire building, alter fire, charcoal
stove
Wood chopping and sawing
Blanket rolls
Menu planning
Outdoor cooking
Garbage disposal
Fishing, hunting, trapping
Construction of three types of
shelter
Camp soil conservation
Crafts from native materials
Lashing

Team Games
Captain Ball
Basketball
Fungo Batting
Hit-pin Baseball
Soccer
Soccer Dodgeball
Volleyball
Softball
Touch Football

Aquatics
Diving
Breast stroke
Advanced skills in all swimming
strokes

Track and Field
50-yard dash
100-yard shuttle relay
Special obstacle relays
Broad jump
Track meet

Elementary Gymnastics
Conditioning and free exercises
Fundamentals for using the back,
horse, Swedish box, single
springboard
Intermediate skill and flying rings
Rope climbing, single and double
ropes

COMPETENCIES TO BE DEVELOPED

What is taught to each age group depends largely upon where
students are on the ladder of their social, emotional, mental, and physical
development as well as the type of handicap each person or subgroup
made up of similar disabilities has. The youngest are often ready for activities usually taught to slightly older children, while retarded 6-year-olds

are more apt to respond to activities thought best for 4-year children. Much experimentation is needed to determine what should be taught. There is a wide gap between the skills that a younger and an older child can do. Devising a list of competencies that should be developed at each age or grade level is wise, and can lead to a better-planned educational program for all age groups. The following list of competencies might well be used as an idea springboard for doing so.

> *General Physical Qualities*
>> Strength
>> Power
>> Endurance
>> Flexibility
>> Agility
>
> *Functional Skill and Coordination*
>> Locomotion (walking, running, skipping, hopping, jumping, climbing, galloping, sliding)
>> Balancing
>> Rhythmic response in movement
>>> Moving to a rhythmic sound
>>> Moving in simple patterns
>>> Skip, slide, polka, schottische, step-hop, waltz, fox-trot, two-step
>>> Patterns—honor, swing, circle, allemande, do-si-do, grand right and left balance, promenade, ladies' chain, right and left through
>> Ball skills
>>> Rolling
>>> Tossing
>>> Throwing—distance and accuracy
>>> Dribbling and juggling
>>> Volleying
>>> Goal shooting
>>> Kicking, dribbling, trapping
>>> Striking—hand, bat, club
>> Rope jumping
>> Beginning swimming
>
> *Creativity, Exploration, and Self-expression*
>
> *Efficient and Attractive Posture*
>> Standing
>> Sitting
>> Moving
>
> *Increasing Emotional Maturity*
>
> *Social Adaptability*

NEED FOR PROGRESSION IN THE PROGRAM

Many believe that today's children are not being challenged or motivated enough educationally. Unfortunately, this is too often true of the physical education program in general and for the handicapped in particular. In the best programs there is both balance and progression through the provision of many types of learning experiences. The use of balls of graduated size, games, dances, and other types of activities that call for many kinds of movement combinations should be stressed. Such progression should be within the many kinds of activities themselves and from grade level to grade level.

THE TEACHING UNIT

A teaching unit is an action blueprint plan devised jointly by the teacher and class. It should be based on the needs of the groups and should provide them with opportunities for growth as individuals and group members. Although there are many ways to organize a teaching unit, basically each should contain a title, an overview or introductory statement, a list of objectives to be reached, an outline of content guides and possible approaches, a list of teacher and learner activities, suggestions for evaluation, and pupil and teacher references. All plans should be kept flexible so that they can be changed, if necessary.

Suggested topics for a unit for sixth-graders in speedball include:

Brief history, nature, and purpose of the game
Soccer skills
  Body traps and blocks
  Dribbling
  Drop kick
  Evading an opponent
  Instep kick
  Kicking for a goal
  Kicking with the inside and outside of the foot
  Passing
  Punting
  Sole-of-foot trap; one-leg trap; two-leg trap
  Tackling
Basketball skills
  Catching and passing
  Overhead juggle
  Pivoting
Speedball skills
  Guarding
  Lifting the ball up to pass
  Pick-up with one foot on a moving ball; on a stationary ball; with two
    feet; with one foot over a moving ball
Rules
  For safety
  For game play
Strategy
Evaluation of skills

THE DAILY ACTIVITY CLASS

Careful planning is basic to good leadership. Although all plans should be flexible, they must be made with a definite purpose to shape all learning experiences to the needs and development of each child *and* to the society of which he is a vital part.

Lesson plans are both time- and energy-savers. They help to assure the building of skill upon skill through a carefully planned and progressively challenging activities program. They also

1. Lead to a faster setting of goals and the attainment of educational, group, and individual objectives
2. Help keep all program offerings in a proper balance so that one area is not overemphasized (such as team relays) to the detriment of another area (such as movement exploration)
3. Make the teacher feel more secure and confident in the leading role
4. Encourage the learner's interest and ability to accept and master greater learning challenges
5. Clarify thought and, through periodic review and practice, help make learning more accurate and permanent
6. Set desirable patterns for students to follow when developing their own study and work habits, as well as when planning their own goals
7. Insure that, during the regular teacher's absence, the substitute leader can carry out previously planned lessons, thus keeping learning continuous
8. Provide for periodic measurement at times that are best for the evaluation of certain kinds of learning results
9. Take into account pupil readiness to move on to new learning experiences
10. Aid in making the best use of each previous activity period for increased pupil learning
11. Help teachers develop and improve teaching skill
12. Can be used as evidence to parents, administrators, and others that educational plans have been devised and that students are being presented new materials

Each lesson should be a meaningful experience in which the pupils learn something new as well as refine previously learned materials and skills. *Build skill upon skill* is a motto recommended for all leaders and most especially for those in charge of physical activities programs.

Class activity plans should include objectives, needed equipment, techniques for linking yesterday's lesson with that of today, new activities to be taught with a time allotment given for each, and ways for evaluating progress.

A well-planned lesson will provide

1. Maximum participation in meaningful activities for all in the group
2. The growth and development of each class member in accordance with stated objectives and desired outcomes
3. Increased pupil interest, appreciation, and enthusiasm for physical activity
4. A variety of activities that have real value and lead toward healthier living for the future as well as the present
5. Opportunities to correlate and integrate physical activities with health and safety measures
6. Opportunities for self-evaluation of student's daily accomplishments

Lesson plans enable the teacher to review and relate to overall program objectives; they serve as a review and help in the preparation of the coming lesson. A good plan provides an organized and progressive procedure that helps maintain class interest and individual motivation. Moreover, it often helps prevent disciplinary problems from arising, as well as helping the teacher to emphasize important points and skill elements. Finally, carefully planned lessons aid in evaluating teacher as well as pupil growth.

THE MIDDLE SCHOOL PROGRAM

Ideally, the sexes should be separated for instruction in physical activity for this age group. Boys tend to be stronger and more skilled in certain activities if they have good coordination and much previous experience in playing games and sports. There are some times, however, when coeducational experiences should be provided for sport skill instruction such as in volleyball, table tennis, or golf, but boys and girls of obviously unequal skills should not be paired nor should any two people who are unequal in capabilities except under unusual learning circumstances (see page 234).

Emphasis should be placed on the mastery of basic sport skills. Lead-up games such as Newcomb for volley-ball, Hit-pin Baseball for softball, or Twenty-one for basketball might well be reviewed before the actual teaching of basic sport skills.

Suggested physical activities for this group include:

Basic Skills in Sports and Games
  Basketball
  Fieldball
  Golf
  Soccer
  Softball
  Skiing
  Speed-a-way
  Speedball
  Tennis
  Touch football
  Track and field
  Volleyball

Dance
  Folk—beginning skills and simple patterns
  Modern dance—basic exercises, movement techniques, simple composition problems
  Social—fox-trot, waltz, and rhumba
  Square—elementary skills and simple figures

Recreational Games
  Active and passive games of low organization
  Archery, tincan, pitch and putt golf

Billiards
Bowling—lawn and duckpin
Carom
Goal shooting
Hiking and camping
Horseshoes
Ice skating
Relays
Roller skating
Table and paddle tennis

Formal Activities and Gymnastics
Beginning fundamental skills on the stationary and flying rings, parallel bars, horse, buck and Swedish box
Body mechanics
Conditioning exercises
Marching

Aquatics
Basic diving skills
Basic swimming strokes
Junior lifesaving
Water games

Stunts and Tumbling
Backward handsprings
Backward roll to handstand
Cartwheels in series
Couple stunts
Dives for distance
Forward and backward rolls
Handsprings
Hand walks
Pyramids
Rebound tumbling
Round offs
Running forward somersaults
Shoulder stand
Stomach balance

In the middle school program, major emphasis should be placed on rigorous physical activity and cooperative group activities. At each grade level the program should include at least four team games, tumbling and gymnastics, track and field events, at least three individual sports, rhythms and dance, as well as first aid and health instruction.

THE HIGH SCHOOL PROGRAM

The high school program should be more advanced, with stress placed upon sports and games, dance, and other areas high in carry-over values for leisure-time use. Coeducational classes should be considered an important part of the program and held at least once weekly. Although most activities included in the offerings may be modified for this purpose and particularly for the handicapped teenager, social and square dancing, volleyball, swimming, tennis, badminton, golf, and bowling can be incorporated with the least amount of difficulty. Such coeducational classes are often best taught jointly by both a man and a woman leader. This is especially true of social dance.

High school students should be given many opportunities to help plan, conduct, and evaluate their program. Stress should be placed on helping them to gain an understanding of the importance of physical activities and fitness, assist each to learn as many leisure-time skills beyond the novice stage, and aid all to build the highest degree of health and strength possible. As future citizens, parents, and community members, those who have enjoyed a meaningful and pleasurable physical activities experience can be great supporters of and believers in a good physical activities program and will be more likely to work toward securing such a program for all age groups in the community, school, and recreation centers throughout the nation.

Suggested activities for the senior high school group include more advanced skills in each of the following areas:

Individual
  Archery
  Badminton
  Bait and fly casting
  Bowling
  Fencing
  Golf
  Handball
  Lead-up games
  Paddle tennis
  Skating, ice and roller
  Skiing
  Squash racquets
  Tennis
  Track and field
  Wrestling

Self-testing Activities
  Acrobatics
  Apparatus
  Gymnastics
  Obstacle course
  Rebound tumbling
  Rope climbing
  Stunts
  Trampoline

Aquatics
  Boating and canoeing
  Diving
  Senior lifesaving
  Skin and scuba diving
  Swimming
  Synchronized swimming

  Water games
  Water safety
  Water ballet

Dance
  Acrobatic
  Folk
  Modern
  Rhythms
  Social
  Square
  Tap

Team
  Baseball
  Basketball
  Field ball for girls
  Field hockey
  Football
  Lacrosse
  Lead-up games
  Soccer
  Speed-a-way
  Speedball
  Touch football
  Volleyball

Formal Activites and Gymnastics
  Body mechanics
  Calisthenics
  Gymnastics
  Marching

Recreational Activities
  Box hockey

Camping and outing	Fly and bait casting
Card games	Games of low organization
Checkers	Hiking
Chess	Horseback riding
Croquet	Horseshoes
Dart ball	Shuffleboard
Duckpins	Yoga

In the high school age group, the program should consist of the refining of skills previously learned and the addition of as wide a variety of individual-dual sports as possible. Coeducational experiences in dance and as many other activities as possible, first aid, and water safety should also be provided.

PHYSICAL ACTIVITY INSTRUCTION FOR OLDER GROUPS

Activities best-suited for older participants include individual sports such as bowling, badminton, and tennis, as well as all types of dancing. Care must be taken so that all taking part in the program gradually build strength, endurance, and overall physical fitness. In the beginning, the instructional and playing time should be short enough that no one will become fatigued. Coed partner play should be emphasized in the racket sports such as table tennis, paddle ball, badminton, and tennis. However, opportunities should also be provided for such separate classes as figure control and handball, for example. Jogging is an ideal activity for those who have medical permission to engage in it.

Senior citizens who have deteriorated and can no longer be independent, whether they are homebound, in nursing homes, or in hospitals, also need a moderate amount of physical activity. Playing games using lighter equipment such as yarn balls or balloons is suggested. Recreational games such as checkers, dominoes, and chess are favorites among this group. However, many persons in this age category are capable of taking care of themselves and are very active physically. Many of the more active ones can enjoy bicycling, hiking, croquet, bowling, social and square dancing. "Leisure villages" and commercial housing projects often supply a variety of activities including medical, housekeeping, shopping, and recreational services. By participating in physical activity programs, older people add zest and good health to their lives. Providing stimulating activities for the aged is an important community responsibility. Great effort should be made to find volunteer leaders within the area to work with this group. Retired teachers and those who love and excel in some sport area are often eager to be of service and feel needed again. Colleges are now increasing the number and kinds of practical experiences students are required to have in order to complete requirements for graduation with a major in any field.

SUGGESTED READINGS

CHAPMAN, FREDERICK, *Recreation Activities for the Handicapped.* New York: Ronald Press, 1960.

KELLY, ELLEN, *Adapted and Corrective Physical Education,* 4th ed. New York: Ronald Press, 1965.

MEYER, HAROLD, CHARLES BRIGHTBILL, and H. DOUGLAS SESSOMS, *Community Recreation,* 4th ed. Englewood Cliffs, N.J.: Prentice-Hall, 1969.

POMEROY, JANET, *Recreation for the Physically Handicapped.* New York: Macmillan, 1964.

RATHBONE, JOSEPHINE, and CAROL LUCAS, *Recreation in Total Rehabilitation.* Springfield, Ill.: Charles Thomas, 1959.

SHIVERS, JAY, and HOLLIS FAIT, *Therapeutic and Adapted Recreational Services.* Philadelphia: Lea & Febiger, 1975.

SMITH, ANNE, *Play for Convalescent Children.* New York: A. S. Barnes, 1961.

VANNIER, MARYHELEN, *Recreation Leadership.* Philadelphia: Lea & Febiger, 1976.

VANNIER, MARYHELEN, MILDRED FOSTER, and DAVID GALLAHUE, *Teaching Physical Education in Elementary Schools,* 5th ed. Philadelphia: W. B. Saunders, 1973.

VANNIER, MARYHELEN, and HOLLIS FAIT, *Teaching Physical Education in Secondary Schools,* 4th ed. Philadelphia: W. B. Saunders, 1975.

13

Active Games and Sports

The contribution the physical activities leader makes as a member of a therapeutic team lies in building the handicapped person's physical strength and endurance; increasing body flexibility; and developing quicker reaction time, as well as speed and accuracy of movement, rhythmic body coordination, body balance, and good posture. This leader must be able to teach his or her students to balance work and play in daily life, to learn the importance of exercise in relationship to health, and to practice good sportsmanship. Many of these ambitious goals can be met by using team sports, modified as necessary according to the disabilities and capabilities of the learners. Team sports can play an important part in helping exceptional people keep physically fit and learn to cooperate with others.

TEAM GAMES AND RELATED SKILLS

Team sports have much to contribute to physical development through large-muscle activities of all those who learn to play and enjoy them. They are especially good for the handicapped, whether they are modified to suit particular movement limitations or are played normally. Being a valued team member is of great importance to everyone, but especially to those who are handicapped. Team games can do much to help disabled individuals gain physical fitness and muscular strength, as well as social skills. Many become challenged to master physical skills in order to keep up with their more active peers and, by so doing, gain added self-confidence as well as greater group acceptance. And those who learn to play team sports often become enthusiastic spectators and avid sports readers.

Organizational Techniques

Because many of the handicapped are lacking in physical skills, teaching them to move their bodies efficiently is basic to all physical education instruction. Drills, relays, and modified team games will motivate further learning in both game skills and cooperative team play.

The instructor should be assisted by helpers; all groups should be kept small for the most effective teaching and learning. Games should be played according to rules whenever possible. Players may be substituted or may interchange duties. A person who can run can go around the bases for a batter who is in a wheelchair in baseball; a student on crutches may help be goalkeeper in soccer with the assistance of a more active team member. Lighter equipment may have to be used.[1] Beep balls and audible goal directionals (as mentioned in an earlier chapter) will help the blind to play team games such as basketball and soccer more skillfully.

Following are some basic team sports that can be taught to the handicapped:

SOCCER SKILLS

Dribble

Tap ball with the inside of the right and left foot alternately, keeping the ball close to the feet and always under control (Figure 13–1). Beginners are apt to kick the ball, then run to catch up.

Passing

Take weight on right foot and swing left leg back and forward, hitting the ball with the inside of the left foot (Figure 13–2). To pass forward left, reverse action, hitting ball with inside of right foot.

Kicking

Swing leg back and contact ball at instep. Keep the toe pointed down (Figure 13–3).

Trapping

Slow balls may be stopped with a raised foot, toes up. As contact is made, the toes are lowered to secure the ball (Figure 13–4). Fast balls are trapped with the leg. If the ball is on the right, take a small step sideways to the left and at the same time roll the right instep in toward the ground and trap the ball with the knee and the inside of the calf.

---

[1] Available from the Cosom Company, Dep't. J., 6030 Wayzata Blvd., Minneapolis, Minn. 55416.

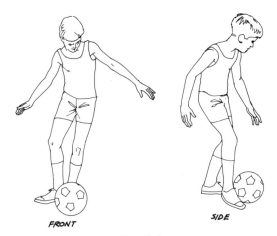

FRONT   SIDE

Fig. 13–1

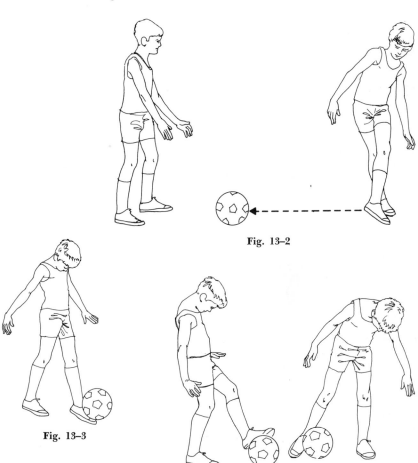

Fig. 13–2

Fig. 13–3

Fig. 13–4

Heading

Get under ball, lower the head slightly, stiffen the neck, and meet the ball with an upward and forward movement to control direction (Figure 13–5). (This skill is too advanced for the majority of elementary children.)

Circle Kick Soccer

Playground, gym
Formation: Single circle, hands joined (Figure 13–6)
Players: 16 to 20
Equipment: Soccerball

1. Ball is rolled into center of circle and players pass the ball around the inside of the circle.
2. Players trap, block, and pass with feet and legs, but keep hands joined.
3. If the ball goes outside the circle, the players between whom it passes are eliminated from the game.
4. When all but five are eliminated, the game is over.

Kick Ball

Playground
Players: 10 to 24
Equipment: Baseball diamond, bases 30 feet apart, soccerball or basketball (Figure 13–7)

1. Seven innings make a game.
2. Pitcher rolls ball to batter, who kicks it into the field.
3. The general rules of baseball apply, with the following exceptions: (a) base runner may be tagged out or "thrown out," (b) runner must be tagged with the ball held in the hand. "Thrown out" means that the base is tagged with the ball or touched by some part of body of baseman or fielder while the ball is in his hands, before the runner reaches base.
4. There may be from 5 to 12 on the team.
5. Use soccerball or basketball.
6. Pitcher's box is 15 to 20 feet from home plate.

Base Football

Playground
Players: 10 to 24
Equipment: Baseball diamond, bases 30 feet apart, soccerball or basketball

1. Kicker punts (kicks from hands) and tries to make all bases without getting put out. May run until ball is held by catcher at home plate or is played to base at which he is running.
2. Score one point if runner completes circuit.
3. Kicker out if (a) ball doesn't go over 10-foot line, (b) ball is caught on fly, (c) touched by ball when in hands of opposing team.
4. Player may stay on base and advance on next kick.
5. Kicking team has 3 outs, then changes places.

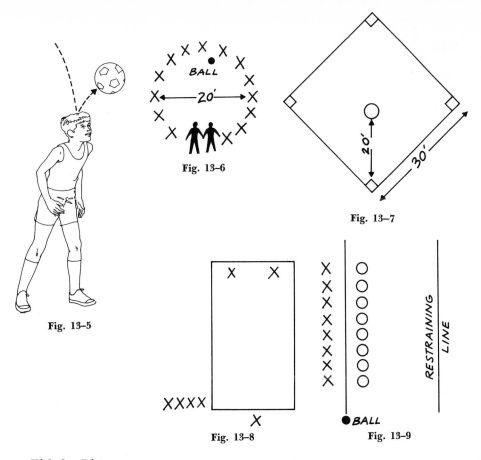

Fig. 13-5

Fig. 13-6

Fig. 13-7

Fig. 13-8

Fig. 13-9

RESTRAINING LINE

BALL

Kick for Distance

Playground
Players: Any number
Equipment: Football, soccerball

1. Line up behind kicking line—two players stand at end of field to recover kicks (Figure 13-8).
2. Each player given definite number of tries.
3. Longest kick recorded—player with longest kick is winner.

Kickover Ball

Playground, gym
Players: 12 to 24
Equipment: Soccerball

1. Players are divided into two teams and placed in parallel lines facing each other (Figure 13-9). Teams alternate putting ball in play.
2. A space is left between the feet of the teams. By superior kicking, one team tries to kick the ball over the heads of the other team.
3. After the ball is kicked over one team's head, the two end players jump up and try to retrieve the ball and run over a restraining line.
4. The team with the most points wins. Game may continue until all get a chance to retrieve the ball.

Line Soccer

Playground: 30′ × 30′ field
Grades: 4–6
Players: Two teams, 8 to 12 players each
Equipment: Soccerball

1. Teams number off and take positions.
2. On signal the soccerball is rolled in from the sideline and the No. 1's on each team run out and try to dribble and kick the ball over the opponent's goal line (Figure 13–10).
3. Guards and linesmen try to stop the ball with feet or hands. If hands are used, the ball must not be held or moved.
4. Score two points for kicking the ball across the opponent's goal line. Score one point for a successful free kick.
5. When one player kicks the ball out of bounds, it is given to the other player in the center of the field.
6. A free kick is awarded for: runner using hands, pushing, blocking, or holding.
7. Free kick: Ball is placed in center of field and player tries to kick it over the opponent's goal line. Neither linesman nor the opposing player must interfere with the kick. Free kick must not pass over goal line.

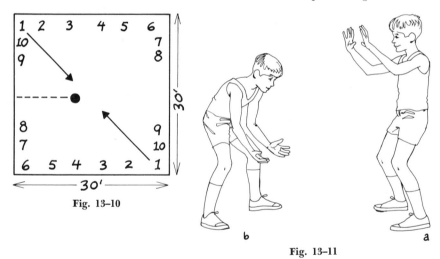

Fig. 13–10

b   a

Fig. 13–11

BASEBALL SKILLS

Catching

Cup relaxed hands, closing firmly when contact is made, and give with the ball. Balls above the waist are caught with fingers up, thumbs together; balls below the waist are caught with hands down, little fingers together (Figure 13–11).

Throwing

UNDERHAND (Figure 13–12a). Hold ball in the hand palm up, weight

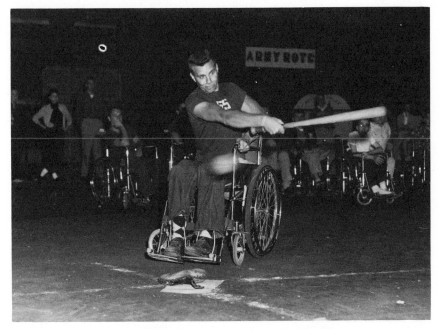

Baseball can be played from a wheelchair. Courtesy of the AAHPER.

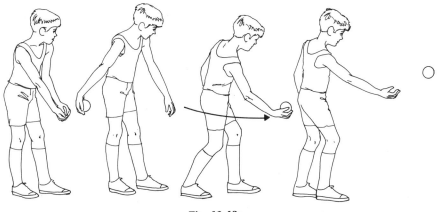

Fig. 13–12a

on the right foot. Swing arm backward, then forward, keeping arm close to body. Simultaneously step forward with the left foot and release the ball at hip level and follow through with weight on right foot. This is a legal pitch.

OVERHAND (Figure 13–12b). Hold ball in hand with palm down and fingers spread easily around the ball. Draw arm backward with elbow bent; swing arm forward using hand, wrist, elbow, and shoulder to deliver ball as weight is shifted to the left foot. Follow through with entire arm and body.

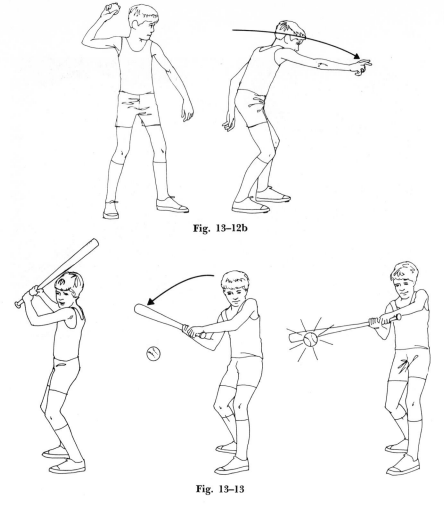

Fig. 13–12b

Fig. 13–13

Batting

Stand facing plate with body parallel to the flight of the ball. Hold the bat in both hands close to the end with right hand on top. Weight is evenly divided on comfortably spread feet, bat is held over the plate, back and at shoulder level. As the pitcher releases the ball, put weight on right foot shifting to left as the bat is swung parallel to the ground. Drop bat and step off on the right foot for the run to first base (Figure 13–13).

Fielding

Stand with feet spread to allow movement in any direction. Ground balls often bounce, so fielder steps forward with fingers down and fields the ball off of his toes (Figure 13–14).

Base Running

Weight is on the left foot as the pitcher starts the throw. Step off on right foot as the pitcher releases the ball or batter gets a hit (Figure 13–15). Run close to the base line and touch each base.

208

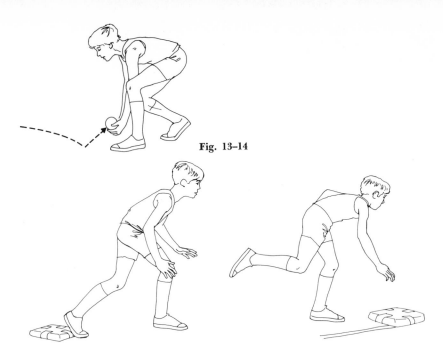

Fig. 13–14

Fig. 13–15

Beat the Ball

Playground, gym
Players: 2 teams
Equipment: Volleyball

1. Play on playground ball diamond (Figure 13–16).
2. Batter throws ball into field and runs the bases; keeps going until he reaches home or is put out.
3. Fielders field ball and throw it to first base; first baseman throws it to second, and on around bases.
4. If runner reaches home before ball does, he scores one point. Otherwise, out.
5. *Variation:* Hand beatball: Same except pitcher pitches ball and batter bats it with open hand.
6. *Variation:* Bowl beatball: Same except pitcher rolls ball and batter kicks it.

Baseball Overtake Contest

Baseball diamond
Players: 8, 12
Equipment: Softball

1. All positions of the infield are occupied except shortstop. Pitcher holds softball.
2. Runner stands on home base and at signal runs the bases (Figure 13–17).
3. At same time, pitcher throws the ball to catcher on home base and from there it is thrown around the bases.
4. One point is scored for each base the runner reaches ahead of the ball.
5. After all members of the running team have run, the teams change positions.

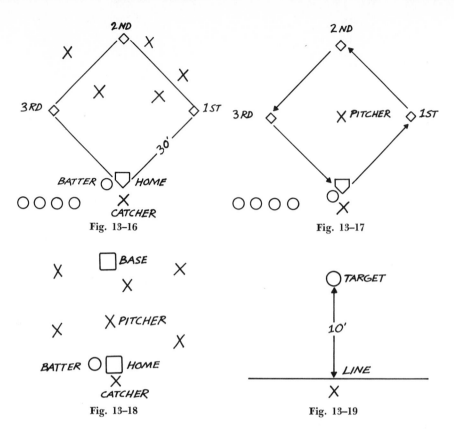

Fig. 13-16

Fig. 13-17

Fig. 13-18

Fig. 13-19

6. Runner throws ball to any player on the opposite team. The fielder throws ball to catcher, etc.

Long Base

Playground
Players: 14, 20
Equipment: Bat and softball

1. Divide into 2 teams.
2. Pitcher throws ball to batter, who bats (Figure 13-18).
3. Runner runs to long base and remains if he arrives before ball.
4. Next runner does same and runner No. 1 comes in.
5. Fielders catch ball and try to put either one out.
6. Runner may make home run if he has time.
7. Out if ball isn't hit in 3 times.
8. When team has 3 outs, change places with other team.

Target

Playground, gym
Players: 8, 12
Equipment: Target, soccerball, or volleyball

1. Target suspended on wall, fence, tree, 10 feet away from thrower (Figure 13-19).

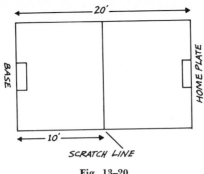

Fig. 13–20

2. Thrower attempts to hit bull's-eye with soccer or volleyball.

3. Each has 3 successive turns and best of three scores is counted.

Bat Ball

Playground, gym (Figure 13–20)
Players: 10, 24
Equipment: Volleyball

1. Divide into two teams, one in field, one at bat.
2. Batter strikes ball with hand or fist. If his hit is successful, he runs to the base, tags it and returns to home plate.
3. A fielder tries to hit the runner. He may only take two steps and can pass the ball to teammates.
4. A player is out when (a) a fly is caught, (b) he is hit by a ball, (c) he does not tag the base, or (d) he does not hit the ball beyond the scratch line. Game may be timed or played by innings. Score 2 points for each complete run and 1 point for a foul made by fielder.

Diamond or Box Ball

Playground
Players: 9 on a team
Equipment: Volleyball

1. "Box" or square made by 3 bases and home base for lower grades. Baseball diamond may be used for upper grades.
2. The pitcher throws the ball so that it bounces once before crossing home plate.
3. The batter strikes the ball with his open hand or clenched fist out into the field. The ball must first strike within the box or diamond for the batter to be safe. If ball strikes outside the diamond, the batter is out.
4. All other baseball rules apply.
5. One point is scored for each successful runner.
6. Nine innings make a game.

Hand Baseball

Playground
Players: 10 on each team
Equipment: Volleyball

1. Use diamond with pitcher 15 feet from home plate.

211

2. Pitcher delivers ball to batter with underhand throw.

3. Batter hits the ball with open hand or fist.

4. A runner may be put out by hitting him with a ball any time he is not on base.

5. Score one for each completed run.

6. Game: Nine innings.

Line Bowling

Playground, gym
Players: 5 on each team
Equipment: Volleyball or softball

1. Two parallel lines, 20′ apart, with boxes at opposite ends from the court (Figure 13–21).

2. Alternate teams try to knock down the pins from their respective boxes.

3. The bowling player on team A replaces the pins in a triangle, 12″ apart, and goes to the foot of his line.

4. Team B player retrieves the ball and bowls from his box.

Progressive Bat Ball

Playground, gym
Players: 10 on a team
Equipment: Volleyball

1. Teams line up in rows directly behind one another (3 to 4 yards apart) with two arms lengths between each player, with their backs to the back line (Figure 13–22).

2. The team farthest from the back line turns and faces the rest.

3. A player tosses a ball and bats it with his hand, then runs to the back line. The ball must go within the square, and the other players attempt to hit the runner before he reaches the line.

4. The runner is out if the ball is caught in the air or if it hits him. If the runner reaches the back line safely, he must return to his team on the next play. Players must maintain their positions and advance the ball by passing only.

5. A batted ball striking outside the square is a foul and the batter is out.

6. One point is scored for each player who reaches the back line and returns to his team.

7. Three outs retires a team which then moves to the back line and the next team in line moves into play.

Race Around the Bases

Playground, gym
Players: Any number to form 2 teams
Equipment: Baseball diamond

1. Two players start from home plate. One player runs to first, second, third, and back to home; the other player runs to third, second, first, and home. Player who reaches home plate first wins.

2. If a player fails to touch a base, he must go back and do so.

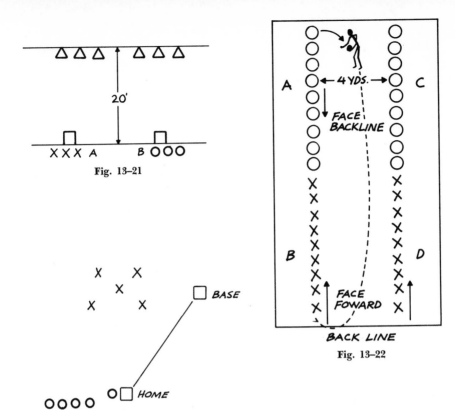

Fig. 13-21

Fig. 13-22

BACK LINE

Fig. 13-23

Throw It and Run

Playground, gym
Players: 10, 18
Equipment: Softball or volleyball

1. Thrower scores run by throwing softball (or rubber volleyball) out into playing field, running to first base and back to home plate (Figure 13-23).
2. If a fielder catches fly ball or returns ball to catcher before thrower returns home, thrower is out.
3. Team scoring most runs wins.

VOLLEYBALL SKILLS

Service

The underhand serve is the simplest to teach, easiest to learn, and most practical for use in placement of the ball. Stand facing opposite court with ball in left hand. Weight is on the right foot as right arm swings backward to shoulder height (Figure 13-24a). Shift weight to left foot as right arm swings forward, knocking the ball out of the left hand (Figure 13-24b). Follow through with the whole body as the ball leaves the right hand (Figure 13-24c). The ball may be struck with the open palm, palm side of the closed fist, or thumb and forefinger side of the closed fist. The assist is generally used in elementary grades.

213

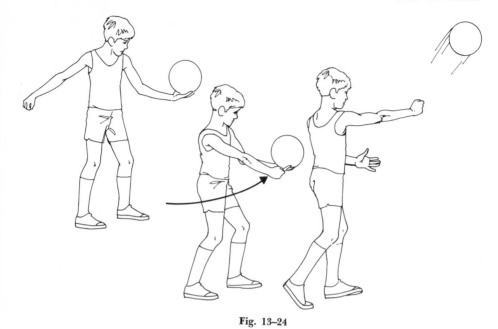

Fig. 13–24

Receiving the Ball

Take a stance with knees slightly flexed. If the ball is high, flex elbows with hands up, take a small step forward, and meet the ball with fingers relaxed (Figure 13–25a). If the ball is low, flex knees more deeply, step forward, and meet the ball with fingers down and palms forward (Figure 13–25b). Children should be taught from the start to keep their eyes on the ball and be ready to receive a volley, or a pass, from a teammate.

Passing the Ball

Try to give upward impetus to the ball and direct it by turning the hands and body toward the desired objective (Figure 13–26). A high ball can be handled more easily and gives a good background for teaching the "set-up" and juggle, which is taught in junior high school.

Rotation

Shake or S-type rotation is used because of its simplicity and the fact that generally 30 to 40 play on each side.

Keep It Up

Playground
Players: Entire class
Equipment: Volley- and basketballs

1. Divide into as many groups as there are volley- and basketball (Figure 13–27).

2. Pitch the ball up in each group and see which group can keep the ball up the longest without it touching the floor.

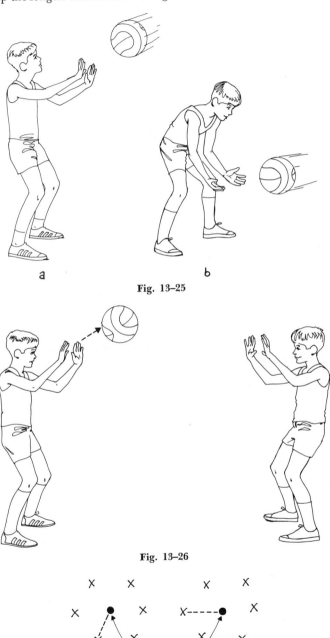

a   b

Fig. 13–25

Fig. 13–26

Fig. 13–27

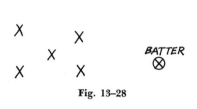

Fig. 13–28

Fig. 13–29

Fist Fungo

Playground, gym
Formation: Scattered (Figure 13–28)
Players: 12, 16
Equipment: Volleyball

1. Batter faces scattered players and bats ball toward them with open hand or fist.
2. A fielder who catches the ball changes place with the batter.
3. A player who fields the ball but does not catch it on the fly tries to hit the batter. The batter may not move his feet.
4. If the batter is hit, he exchanges places with the fielder. If he is not hit, he has another turn.

Cage Ball

Playing field: 30 to 80 feet, according to age groups
Players: 10 to 50
Equipment: Large ball and volleyball net

1. The net is placed at 8 feet, and the area is marked into 3 playing divisions (Figure 13–29).
2. Each player must stay within assigned area.
3. The server stands back of the line and tosses or bats the ball to a player, who assists it over the net.
4. Players rotate for service, and only the serving team can score.
5. When the ball is not assisted on service, is dropped, goes into net, or out of bounds, it goes to the opposing team.

Shower Ball

Playing field: out of doors or inside
Players: Any number to form 2 teams
Equipment: Volleyball and net

1. Ball may be batted or tossed over the net.

2. Only one player on each side may handle the ball, and it cannot be held over 3 seconds. A player may only take one step with the ball.

3. Points are given for violations and each time the ball touches the ground.

Newcomb

Playing field: Tennis court or volleyball court
Players: Any number to form 2 teams
Equipment: Volleyball or soccerball and net

1. The ball is thrown back and forth over the net, and team members attempt to keep it from touching the ground on their side.

2. Any number of players may handle a ball on one side, but it must not be held over 3 seconds.

3. A point is scored when the ball touches the ground or goes out of bounds.

BASKETBALL SKILLS

Stance

Stand with feet apart, knees slightly bent to permit shifts in all directions.

Passing

Concentrate on accuracy, passing with just enough momentum so that the ball may be caught easily. Step in the direction of the pass in order to back up teammates (Figure 13–30).

OVERHEAD TWO-ARM. Arms above head, elbows slightly bent (Figure 13–31a). Propel ball straight forward (Figure 13–31b).

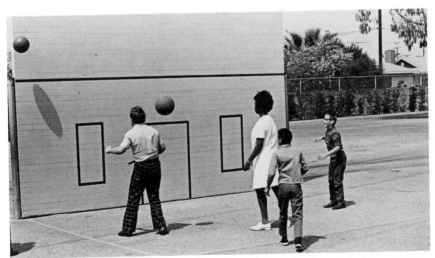

A backboard can help one learn throwing and catching skills more quickly. Courtesy of the Los Angeles Public Schools.

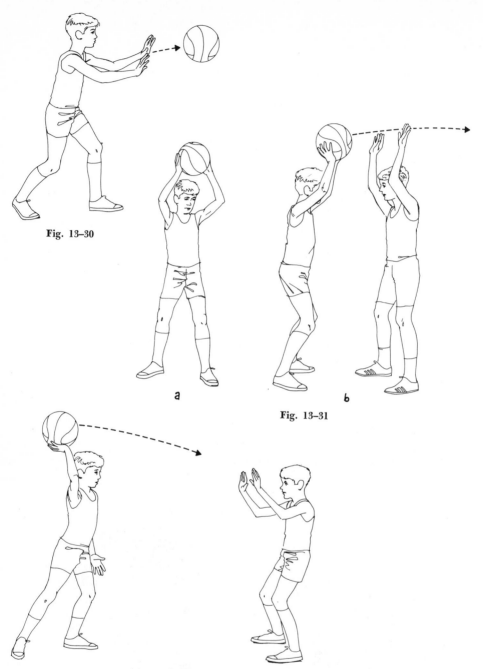

Fig. 13–30

a

Fig. 13–31

b

Fig. 13–32

OVERHEAD ONE-ARM. Same as above, except ball is balanced on one hand (Figure 13–32).

CHEST. Ball is held to chest with elbows bent. Push ball forward and upward as arms are extended, and release when arms are straight (Figure 13–33).

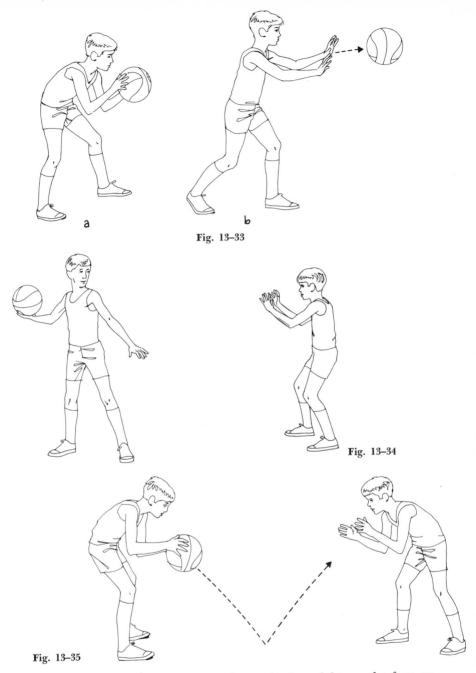

Fig. 13–33

Fig. 13–34

Fig. 13–35

SIDE-ARM. Balance ball on hand, arm back, weight on the foot on the same side. Transfer weight to other foot as ball is thrown (Figure 13–34).

BOUNCE. Arms in position as for chest pass (Figure 13–35). Keep ball low, because high bounces are easily intercepted. Ball is held to side, one arm across chest, both elbows bent. Throw ball as arms are extended.

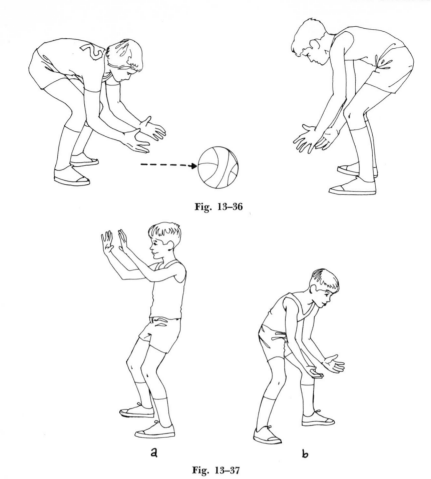

Fig. 13–36

a   b

Fig. 13–37

ROLL PASS. Allow children who have not advanced far in skills to roll the ball on the floor as in bowling (Figure 13–36).

Catching

Receive high balls with fingers up, low balls with fingers down. Relax hands and give with the ball. Always keep eye on the ball.

Shooting Baskets

ARCH. Hold ball slightly to the front about chin level, with fingers up, elbows bent. Look at the basket, straighten arms, and push the ball in a high arch (Figure 13–38).

LAY-UP SHOT. Player receives ball under or close to basket, jumps into air, and tries to lay the ball so that it will enter just over the rim of the basket (Figure 13–39).

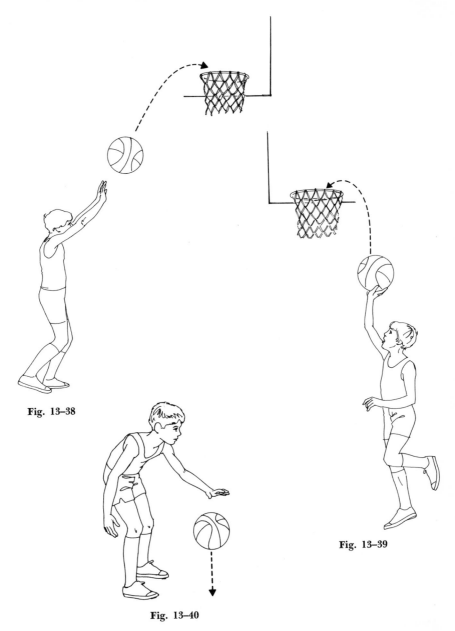

Fig. 13–38

Fig. 13–39

Fig. 13–40

DRIBBLE. Body is in crouch position, head up so that the player can look over the court. Bounce the ball low by flexing the wrist back and hitting the ball with the fingers (Figure 13–40). (Elementary-grade children do not develop a high degree of skill in dribbling because they lower their heads to watch the ball.)

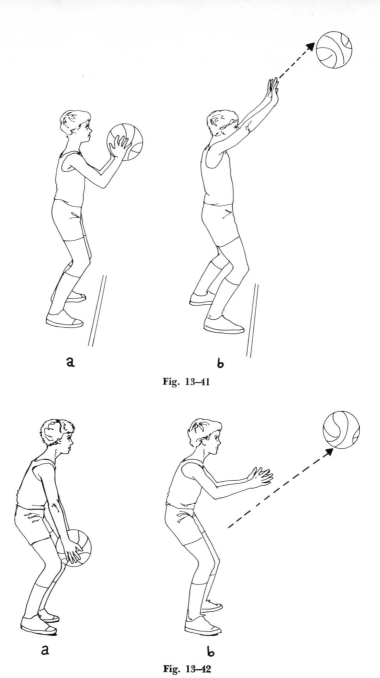

a   b

Fig. 13–41

a   b

Fig. 13–42

Foul Shots

ARCH. Same as high arch shot, but knees are flexed more (Figure 13–41a) and toes must not cross the foul line (Figure 13–41b).

SCOOP. Small children find it easier to shoot a foul shot by catching the ball with fingers down (Figure 13–42a) and throwing it underhanded in a high arch (Figure 13–42b).

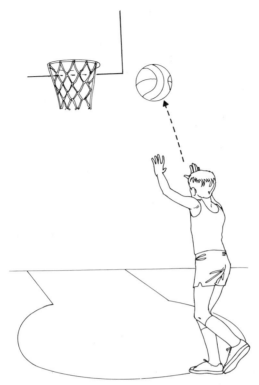

Fig. 13–43

Twenty-One

Basketball court
Players: 2 to 12
Equipment: Basketball

1. Players take a long shot (15 to 20 feet) and a short shot at the basket (Figure 13–43).
2. Long shot scores 2 points and short shot 1 point.
3. Players take turns and the first to score 21 points wins.
4. *Variation:* Players may shoot from the foul line, retrieve the ball, and take a short shot. Small, light ball may be used for younger children.

Catch, Throw, and Sit

Gym
Players: 8 to 12 on a team
Equipment: Basketballs

1. Divide group into teams of 8 to 12. Line up against walls of gym or in a hollow square.
2. Captain faces his team and stands 15 feet from them; he must keep one foot in a 3-foot circle.

3. At signal, captain throws ball to first player on right, who catches it, throws it back and then sits down. This is repeated down the line.
4. If any player or captain fails to catch the ball, he must recover it and return to position before throwing it.
5. Team which has all players seated first wins.

Keep Away

Playground, gym
Players: 8
Equipment: Baseball or basketball

1. Draw court of four rectangles about 6 by 10 feet.
2. Place 2 pupils in each rectangle.
3. Those in alternate rectangles are partners; they try to keep the ball away from the other two.
4. When a player steps on or out of the line, the ball goes to the opposite team.

Sideline Basketball

Basketball court
Players: 2 teams
Equipment: Basketball

1. Two members of each team play on the floor and the rest of the players line up on the side.
2. Regulation basketball rules are followed, except the ball may be passed to teammates on the sidelines.
3. Both teams play the same basket.
4. The defensive team becomes offensive by throwing the ball to a player on the sidelines.
5. The center line is out of bounds, and stepping over any line gives the ball to the opposing team on its sideline.
6. Ball may be put into play by center toss or by giving the ball on the sidelines to the team scored against.
7. Players on sidelines rotate with players on floor.
8. Score 2 points for each basket made and 1 point for free throw after a foul.

Keyhole Basketball

Area around basket
Players: 2 to 10
Equipment: Basketball

1. Chalk eight marks around basket (Figure 13–44).
2. No. 1 player shoots from the first mark.
3. If he makes the basket, he moves on and shoots from the No. 2 mark and on around until he misses.
4. The other players shoot in turn and advance counterclockwise.
5. The first player who reaches his original position wins.

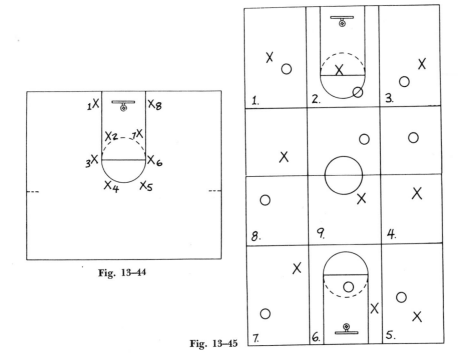

Fig. 13–44

Fig. 13–45

Nine-Court Basketball

Basketball court divided into 9 equal areas (Figure 13–45)
Players: Two teams of 9 each
Equipment: Basketball

1. Play as basketball except each player is assigned an area and must stay within that boundary.
2. Players advance the ball toward their goal by passing; they may dribble one time. Only forwards may shoot at the goal.
3. Ball is put in play by a center toss.
4. Unguarded free shot, worth 1 point, is awarded for fouls (blocking, holding, etc.).
5. Ball is taken out of bounds for infractions (such as crossing line, traveling, etc.).

Active Team Games for Young Children

Children as well as adults like to play games that are simple, fast-moving, and fun. Many young children's games are ideal for both the mentally retarded and those who have had limited opportunity to learn such simple activities as Red Light or Squirrel in the Trees.

The interest span of very young children is short. The leader can best work with this group by introducing several new games during an allotted time rather than only using one or two. A new game should be started when interest in the current activity starts to lag. Other suggestions that may be helpful in beginning to develop the interest of young disabled children in team activities are:

1. Give directions as simply and accurately as possible.
2. Demonstrate as you describe how the game is played.
3. Get each game started as quickly as possible.
4. Choose games best suited to the needs, interests, and abilities of the group.
5. Rotate often the opportunities to be "It."
6. Let children gradually develop their own leadership.
7. Remember that those on the fringe of a crowd will voluntarily join a group that is having great fun. Forcing the child to play is usually wasted effort.
8. Create an air of expectancy. It will aid in keeping group control.
9. Talk quietly to your group. Shouting only encourages more noise and confusion.
10. Discover your own best method for getting the group to listen to your directions. Some people use a whistle, piano chord, or upraised or clapped hands to get attention.
11. Play with the group.

Children of ages 5 to 10 will find delight in the following team activities.

SIMPLE GROUP GAMES

Catch a Fish

Players divide into two teams—the fish and the net. Each group stands behind a goal line—50 to 75 feet apart and parallel. Players of one group join hands to form the net. On a signal, both groups move forward, the fish trying to reach the other goal. Fish can only go around ends. Net must make circle around the fish. Those caught are out of the game. This continues till all are caught. Then teams reverse.

Old Mother Witch

One player is witch and walks in front of the group. Players follow, calling, "Old mother witch fell in the ditch. Picked up a penny and thought she was rich." Witch turns around and asks the leader of the group, "Whose children are you?" Leader says any name, and they start again, but if the response is "Yours," the witch chases the children. The first child caught is the new witch. Or the witch catches as many as possible and then chooses a new witch.

Catch the Caboose

Form groups of four in line, each clasping arms around the player in front. The last in line is the caboose, and the head player is the engine.

"It" tries to hook on to the last player, while each line tries to prevent this. If "It" succeeds in hooking onto the file, the first in line becomes the new "It" and tries to join another line. Several "Its" add interest to the game. Begin with one and add the others gradually.

Flowers and the Wind

Divide into two equal groups, with home bases at opposite sides of the room. One group is the wind. The other group represents different flowers—two or three of each kind. Flowers advance and play near home of the wind. Wind tries to guess what flowers they are. As soon as the right name is said, the flowers of that name run home with the wind chasing them. Any players caught join the winds. Remaining flowers repeat their play, continuing till all flowers are caught.

Run for Your Supper or The Flying Dutchman

Form circle and join hands. One person is "It" and stands outside. "It" touches hands of two players and says, "Run for your supper." The two players take off, running in opposite directions (always passing on the right side). "It" takes place of one runner. Whichever of the two runners fails to get back in first is new "It."

Fox Trail

Make a circle 15 to 30 feet in diameter with spokes and a smaller second circle of about 10 feet inside. "Dens" are on the spoke line. Hunter takes position in center den circle. Foxes run to dens—but one fox has no den. Foxes try to change dens (on signal) without being caught by the hunter. Odd player tries to get a den. All must stay on the lines. Any player tagged by the hunter (any time he is out of a den) becomes a hunter. Several hunters add interest.

Red Light

Two parallel lines are drawn 50 to 75 feet apart to mark the playing field. "It" stands in the center of the field with his back to the group. Other players are on the line behind him. "It" counts to ten and calls out, "No talking, no laughing, no moving. Red Light." On "Red Light," he faces the group. During counting, the other players go as far toward the opposite line as possible, but must stop and obey "It's" command. "It" sends those he sees moving back to the starting line and counts over again. First one to reach opposite line becomes "It" for the next game.

Midnight

Markings: Two long lines at end of room parallel and 3 feet apart. At opposite end—50 to 75 feet away—another line is drawn parallel to these. Fox stands behind the double lines. Mother hen and her chicks stand in front of the double lines. Mother hen asks the fox, "What time is it, Mr. Fox?" He might answer any hour, but if he says "Midnight," the hen and chicks must run to the other end of the room. Those caught become foxes. Only the Old Fox answers the hen's question. Game continues until all are caught. Last child becomes the fox for the next game. If hen is caught another is chosen.

Animal Blind Man's Buff

One blindfolded player stands in center of circle with a cane or stick. All the players skip around in a circle until "It" taps three times with the cane. All stand still. "It" points to a player who then takes the opposite end of the cane in his hand. "It" asks him to make a noise like a cat, dog, cow, sheep, lion, parrot, duck, etc. "It" tries to guess who the other player is. If correct, "It" goes to the circle and the other player takes his place. If wrong, he is "It" again.

Animal Chase

Two pens are on opposite corners of playground. One player is called a "chaser." Other players make teams, calling themselves by animal names—two or three of each kind—all in one pen. Chaser calls out animal names (one at a time). All animals of that name run to reach other pen before the chaser catches them. The one caught takes the chaser's place and the game continues.

Frog in the Pond

The frog sits with crossed feet. All players circle around him. Players tease him while chanting, "Frog in the middle, can't catch me." The frog, who must remain seated, tries to tag the rest. The tagged player becomes the new frog and the old one joins the circle. Add two or more frogs as the players become more skillful.

BALL GAMES

Tether Ball (A two or more person game)

Tie a tennis ball in a sock or net and attach it to a long heavy cord suspended from a pole 10 to 13 feet long. Two players, each with a tennis racket or paddle tennis racket, alternate hitting the ball while standing at opposite sides of the pole. Each must stay in his own area and try to hit the ball to wind it completely around the pole above the 6-foot mark. The server may hit the ball in any direction. His opponent must always hit it in the opposite direction. A point is scored when the ball rests against the pole above the mark. The point is given to the player in whose direction the cord is wound. Alternate serves after each point. Play for ten points. As many as four can play this game with two on each team.

Throw It and Run

The throwers line up in single file to one side of home plate. The fielders arrange themselves in a semicircle in the field. To begin the game, one of the throwers steps to home plate and throws the ball out into the playing field. He then runs to first base and back home. The game continues until all the throwers have been at bat. Then the throwers become fielders. A person is out if the fielders catch the ball on the fly or throws it to the catcher at home plate before the thrower gets back home.

Kick It and Run

Play is similar to "Throw It and Run," except the throwers are kickers. A pitcher is used by the fielders and the ball is kicked rather than thrown. Three fouls (outside the boundaries) constitute an out.

Double Circle Ball

Two circles are formed. Each side has a volleyball or basketball. Players in each circle throw the ball to anyone on their team. Score a point each time the ball is caught. The winning team is the one that scores the most points in three minutes.

End Dodgeball

All players form circle except six players, who line up, hands on hips of next person—all inside the circle. Players forming circle pass ball around and toss it, trying to hit the player at the end of the line. Player is out when he is hit. When one is left, choose another six. Head man in lines moves around facing person who holds ball—as quickly as he can move. All try to keep end man from being hit.

Indian Club Guard Ball

Team A forms as small a circle as possible around three upright Indian clubs—team faces outward. Team B, facing inward, makes an outer circle about 10 feet away. Team B tries to knock over the clubs with volleyballs or basketballs. Teams change places when all three clubs are down.

Center Base

All players but one form circle, 20 feet in diameter. "It" stands in center, throws ball to a player, and immediately runs out of the circle. Player catches ball, returns it to the center of the circle or a marked spot, and then chases "It." "It" can be saved only by touching the ball. Running must be near the circle. "It," when caught or saved, chooses another "It" and the game starts over.

STUNTS

Catch the Cane

All stand in a circle except "It." All have numbers. "It" stands a cane on the floor with one finger on top, then calls a number and raises finger from the cane. Number called must catch cane before it hits the floor. He is "It" if he succeeds.

Follow the Leader

Leader starts any activity (jump, roll, hop). All must follow. Those missing must go to the end of the line. Second person in line starts an activity, etc.

Alphabet

Two teams have cards with letters of alphabet; each player holds one. All line up facing a line drawn halfway between the teams. "It" calls a simple word (using letters players hold), and players with letters rush to the line and spell the word with the cards. First side to get it right wins.

Jump the Shot

All players but one form a circle. Odd player holds one end of a rope and swings it around so that a weight attached to the other end skims the ground. Other players jump over the rope as it swings past them. Any player who fails to jump over the rope is eliminated.

Three-Legged Box Race

Two groups of three compete. Numbers one and three of each group stand with each foot in a box. Player two has one foot in each of their boxes. Players advance by scooting boxes forward, being careful not to step out of the boxes. Team crossing finish line first wins.

Bean Roll

Form two teams. Give first players in line a bean and a toothpick. Each must roll his bean to the end line. The team that finishes first wins.

LEAD-UP TEAM GAMES FOR CHILDREN

Children need to learn certain basic movement skills. These include such simple skills as learning how to kick, throw, and dodge a ball. Ball technique games include the following:

Ball Toss

Playground, playroom, gym
Formation: Circle
Players: 8 to 12
Equipment: Large ball

1. Ball is thrown around circle.
2. Player in center throws to each player in circle, who returns ball to thrower (Figure 13–46).
3. Concentrate on throwing and catching; as skill improves, increase speed.

Boundary Ball

Gym, playground
Players: 20 to 40
Equipment: Volleyball or soccerball

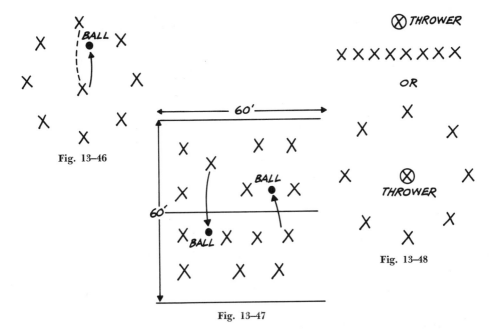

Fig. 13–46

Fig. 13–47

Fig. 13–48

1. Draw two parallel lines 60 feet long and 60 feet apart. Draw a center line.
2. Divide players evenly and place teams at opposite ends of the field facing center (Figure 13–47).
3. The line in back of each team is that team's goal.
4. At a given signal each team tries to throw a ball across the other team's goal line.
5. Players try to keep opponents' ball from crossing the goal.
6. Team that gets the ball across goal first wins.

Call Ball

Playground, gym
Formation: Line or circle (Figure 13–48)
Players: 8 to 12
Equipment: 8″ rubber ball or volleyball

1. One player is thrower.
2. Thrower calls name of a player and tosses ball in the air.
3. Player whose name is called attempts to catch the ball. If he succeeds, he changes places with the thrower.
4. If a player misses, the thrower calls names until the ball is caught.
5. In a new and unacquainted group, number off and call a number, or call colors of clothing.

Circle Kick Ball I

Gym, playground
Formation: Circle (Figure 13–49)
Players: 18 to 30, number off by twos to form teams

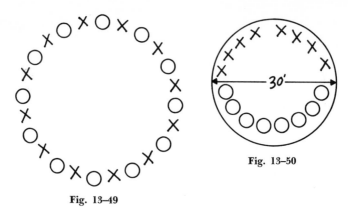

Fig. 13–50

Fig. 13–49

1. Each player attempts to kick ball between the legs of two opposing players. Score one point for a successful kick.
2. If a player kicks the ball over the heads of the opposing team, the opponents score a point.

Circle Kick Ball II

Gym, playground
Formation: Circle (Figure 13–50)
Players: 16 to 24, two teams, two captains
Equipment: Rubber volleyball

1. Ball is put in play by being kicked toward opponent.
2. While the ball is in play all players must stay in their half of the circles. Only captains may move out of position to kick balls that have stopped out of teammates' reach.
3. One point is scored for a team each time player kicks ball through opponents' half-circle; player kicks ball out over shoulders; opponent kicks ball out on his own side; or opponent plays ball with hands.
4. Player who receives the ball when it goes out puts it into play again.

Circle Club Bowls

Playground, gym
Formation: Circle
Players: 12 to 24
Equipment: Indian clubs, softball, volleyball

1. Form a circle. Place a club in back of each player, who stands in stride position (Figure 13–51).
2. Each player tries to throw the ball through the legs of another player.
3. Player whose club is knocked down is out of the game.

Hot Ball

Gym, playground, playroom
Formation: Circle or double line (Figure 13–52)
Players: 12 to 20
Equipment: Any kind of ball

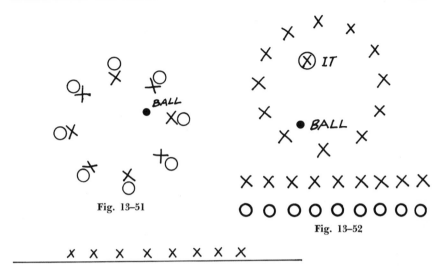

Fig. 13–51

Fig. 13–52

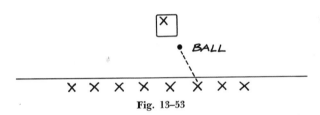

Fig. 13–53

1. Players pass ball as rapidly as possible around circle. Players who drop ball must drop out of game.
2. *Variation 1:* "It" in center of circle may try to touch the ball as it is passed from one player to the next. If he succeeds, he changes place with the player who had the ball when it was touched.
3. *Variation 2:* Group forms double lines facing each other. On signal, balls are passed to the end of the line and back. The line finishing first wins.

Line Dodgeball

Gym, playroom, playground
Players: 12 to 24
Equipment: Volleyball

1. Two lines are drawn about 20 feet apart. Halfway between lines a box about 4 feet square is drawn.
2. One player stands in the box. Half the players stand on one line and half on the other (Figure 13–53).
3. Players on both lines take turns throwing and trying to hit the center player below the waist.
4. The center player may dodge but must never have both feet out of the box at any time. If hit, the center player changes places with the person who threw the ball.

skilled players should be on each team. Using the couple-partner method of grouping, those in wheelchairs can bat the ball and have their partners run the bases for them. With this pairing method, even blind children can be taught to do such things as swim, dive, and roller skate if guided by a sighted person.

INDIVIDUAL ACTIVITIES

Individual sports can be played alone or with a partner or opponent. There are many popular sports activities for both normal and handicapped persons. They can be enjoyed almost throughout life; they also increase good health, vigor, and physical fitness, and provide opportunities for competition. They are particularly valuable in providing the chance for people to channel hostilities and aggressions constructively.

Almost any individual sport can be enjoyed by the handicapped if it is modified. Horseshoes, ring toss, kite flying, marbles, table tennis, shuffleboard, and tether ball are highly recommended. Other excellent sports are horseback riding [3] and fishing. In this section, the basic ac-

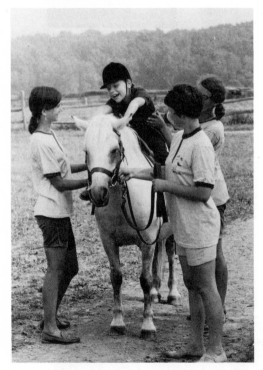

Riding is a great adventure for all would-be cowboys! Courtesy of the National Foundation for Happy Horsemanship for the Handicapped, Inc.

[3] Write to Maudie Warfel, The National Foundation for Happy Horsemanship for the Handicapped, Box 462, Malvern, Pennsylvania, for excellent materials on teaching horsemanship.

tivities and skills of archery, badminton, bowling, golf, tennis, and swimming are listed. Some suggestions are also provided for adaptations of each of these sports for handicapped people. But, as has been mentioned before, the teacher must use his or her own knowledge of the particular disabilities of the learners. These sports will be only sketchily discussed to give the reader a general idea of the basic movements and skills involved in teaching them to people with various types of disabilities.

In teaching any activity, one should make sure that there is enough needed equipment for each student. Instruction should be given in small groups. In some cases, handicapped and normal students can be placed in the same classes, especially if one who is skilled is paired with a handicapped beginner. Lighter equipment is often best for the latter, especially in bowling, archery, and tennis. Bowling skills and scoring methods can be taught with sets of polyethylene pins and balls, and even with Indian clubs, sand-weighted milk cartons used as bowling pins, and volleyball or small playground balls as bowling balls.

Bowling alleys, archery ranges, golf courses and/or driving ranges, and municipal pools can often be used free or for a nominal charge during off hours. Some establishments will even furnish instruction.

The teacher should see that the program gains publicity in school or local newspapers, through bulletin-board displays, etc. Awards should be given to all participants who earn them. Tournaments add interest, as well as giving motivation both to participants and spectators.

ARCHERY

For the handicapped and/or beginners, shooting at shorter distance is recommended. It is especially important in these cases that the target area be level. Individual assistance should be given to orient the blind to the location of the target and the anchor position on the face. Each should get the "feel" of the target size and each scoring ring. For indoor archery, lighter equipment can be used; arrows with suction cups can be shot at cardboard wall targets.

Necessary equipment for archery includes bows, arrows, targets, arm guards, and shooting tabs or gloves. Archery is a skill that can be performed by many handicapped people. It requires a use of the arms and eyes in particular. Even wheelchair victims are able to enjoy this sport if it is adapted to their abilities.

BADMINTON

Badminton is a net game requiring eye-hand coordination that can be played as a singles or doubles game with one or two players on a side. The object is to hit the bird or shuttlecock away from the opponent but inside the playing area. This game involves less strength than coordination, and so is an excellent choice for those disabled people who are less strong.

A match consists of the best of three games. Players change ends at the start of the second game, and if needed, also at the third game. In

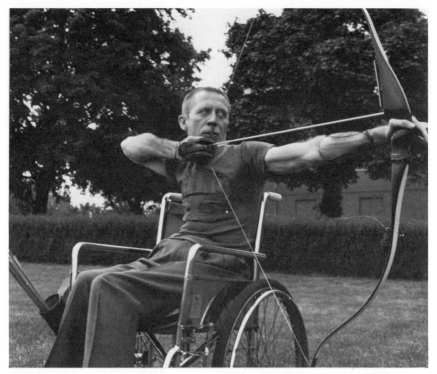

Archery is one of the best sports for many of the handicapped, for it is a lifetime sport and can be played indoors as well as outside. Courtesy of the AAHPER.

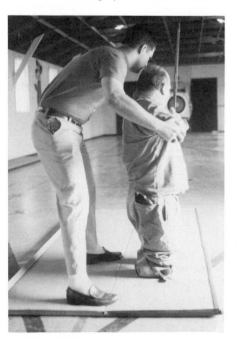
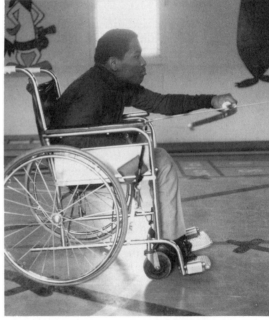

Archery is an ideal camp activity. Courtesy of the AAHPER and the National Wheelchair Athletic Association.

the third game, players change sides when the first player reaches 8 in a game of 15 points, or 6 in a game of 11 points.

For handicapped people, three players can be on each side when the basic strokes are being taught. Games can be played for fewer points to win until the students gain an understanding of the game. You can teach badminton inside, for it is often too difficult for students to control the bird when playing outside. If this is impossible, you can use heavier, weighted birds.

BOWLING

Bowling is one of the best activities for the handicapped of almost all ages and types. It is easily learned, although playing well and scoring consistently high is a difficult but obtainable challenge. The various techniques can be adapted and taught according to the capabilities of the individuals involved. This is a game that requires practice and skill, but it gives the handicapped an excellent chance to socialize, compete, and have fun while improving their physical skills.

For those in wheelchairs, the chair should face the pins squarely and the bowler should take two or more preliminary swings before releasing the ball. Blind students should walk the width and length of the alley, feel how the pins are arranged, and be aided in selecting a ball best suited for each one. A wooden waist-high frame can be used to guide the bowler to the best place to stand (as set by a sighted assistant) in order to make a strike and pick up spares. Braille score sheets can be made or purchased commercially.[4] Small children and those who lack

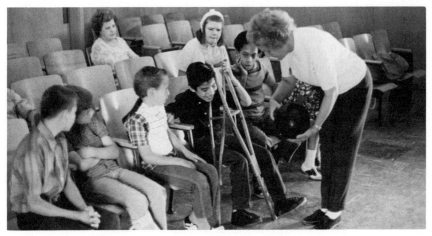

The teacher should "show" as well as "tell" how to select just the right kind of a bowling ball. Courtesy of the Los Angeles Public Schools.

---

[4] For more information concerning products available for teaching the blind to bowl, write to the National Society For The Prevention of Blindness, 1790 Broadway, New York, 10019.

arm strength should use lighter polyethylene balls and pins. Those without arms can use their feet to roll or push the ball forward.

GOLF

Needed equipment for golf includes clubs, tees, balls, golf bags, a golf course or driving range. An indoor area may be substituted, but here plastic or cotton balls should be used instead of regular ones; the balls may be hit off rubber mats.

TENNIS

Needed equipment includes rackets and balls. The game may be played inside or outside.

Tennis is a good activity for those who are not blind or confined to crutches or a wheelchair. Even one-armed persons can play the game by tossing the ball up off the face of the racket on the serve. Although the cerebral palsied have difficulty learning the strokes, and especially the serve, with great patience and perseverence, many do learn to play fairly well. Hitting the ball on a backboard is recommended until one gets the rhythm of the various strokes. Short and lighter rackets are suggested for younger players and those lacking in physical strength.[5]

SWIMMING

Because swimming is one of the best physical activities for the handicapped of all ages, more space will be devoted to describe it than the other individual and paired activities, such as bowling, tennis, etc. This skill enables people with disabilities to perform a wider range of movements than they could do otherwise. It also helps them to relax, gain self-confidence, and learn recreational skills for their own enjoyment. It is an excellent way of sharing recreational experience with others, and it teaches people safety skills for their own protection. As a recreational therapist for Pacific State Hospital in Pomona, California has pointed out:

> Swimming provides the first real step to rehabilitation because it has something for everyone. An aquatic program can include non-ambulatory, severely retarded, and others whose recreational opportunities and experiences might otherwise be limited. Swimming success—whether achievement of swimming skills or simply adjustment to the water—may motivate an individual to try other activities.[6]

Class organization. The size of a swimming class depends upon the handicap of the participants. If their disabilities are mild, some might

---

[5] For sources of this kind of equipment see the appropriate issues of the *Journal of Health, Physical Education, and Recreation.*

[6] Frances Grove, "Aquatic Therapy: A Real First Step to Rehabilitation," *Programs for the Handicapped* (Washington, D.C.: AAHPER, October 1970).

well be included in a class with normal students. For those with more severe handicaps such as marked retardation or complete blindness, instruction must be on a one-to-one basis; the teacher will need the assistance of others. The teacher and the helpers must completely understand each student's physical problem, movement range, or other limitations. They must also know the kinds of movements each learner needs to learn to make in order to gain maximum therapeutic benefit.

Safety Precautions. All safety precautions must be taken at all times. Each student should be required to wear a plastic safety bubble or inflated water rings until the instructor can assess the ability of each person for grouping and instructional purposes. Nonswimmers should be required to wear such devices at all times while in the water. Strict safety rules such as no running on the deck, no horseplay in the water, etc. should be clearly understood by everyone before instruction begins. Special techniques for getting in and out of the pool should be taught first, for doing so helps beginners to gain feelings of security. Ramps, handrails, widely spaced steps, and other types of safety equipment should be provided. Long floating cork ropes should divide the pool into its shallow and deeper parts. It is imperative that the teacher be able to see each student; and unless the students are blind, all should be able to see her.

Preliminary Skills. The water in which beginners are taught must be warm (82 to 84 degrees). A child or adult who is cold and shivering will become tense and learn little. Splashing of wrists, arms and back

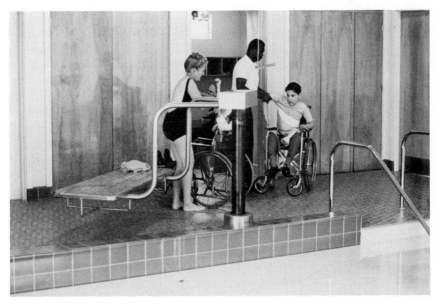

Some children will need much assistance in order to enter the pool. Courtesy of the Los Angeles Public Schools.

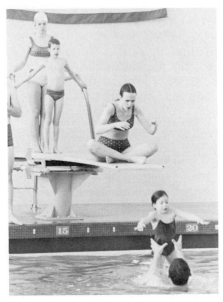

Swimming instruction for many of the handicapped should be on a one-to-one basis. Courtesy of the Wisconsin State University.

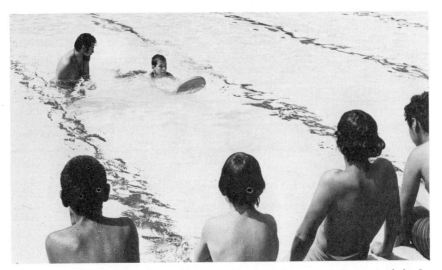

The use of flutter boards can help some learners feel more secure. Courtesy of the Los Angeles Public Schools.

of neck breaks the shock of entry. Jumping up and down helps increase circulation. The most important task for the instructor is to build the pupil's self-confidence—thus he or she must have both confidence in you as an instructor and confidence in his own ability to learn. At this point, there can be no hurry, and play must be mixed freely with instruction. Keep in mind the attention span of your charges and remember that confidence and relaxation are of prime importance.

Following are some water skills that can be taught to the handicapped:

Ducking—Hold gutter with one hand and nose with the other. Squat and submerge head.

Breath-Holding—Compare the chest to a balloon. Demonstrate by gasping in breath and showing that the air is held in the chest cavity and not in puffed-out cheeks. Hold breath above water and later submerge.

Opening Eyes—Hold breath, submerge, and open eyes under water. Count fingers or pick up toys or pebbles from the bottom. This not only gives confidence but eliminates the habit of wiping water from the eyes, which slows up teaching.

Exhaling—Not being able to breathe is terrifying, so breath control is of utmost importance. Exhalation should be easy and relaxed. Forcing the breath out through the mouth and nose under pressure, as if blowing out a candle, hurries the process at first; later the exhalation more nearly resembles a sigh. Hold the gutter for the first trials. Later, stand in shallow water, bend at the waist, and repeat inhaling and exhaling five times in succession.

Bobbing—Inhale above the water, submerge with knees flexed, and exhale. Shoot the body above water and repeat. This is fun and gives excellent practice in rhythmic breathing. This technique is used later as a safety device in progressing from deep to shallow water.

Relaxing—Take a deep breath, bend at the waist, and drop head into water. Let arms hang loosely and allow knees to buckle.

Prone Float—Place fingertips lightly on the gutter, take a breath, submerge face, and stay under water long enough to allow feet to float to top. Tap gutter four or five times with fingers.

Tuck Float—Once the learner has learned to relax, he should be assured that the water will support his body. There are a few who cannot float easily because of weight displacement (wiry, lean children rather than the well-padded ones), but propulsion of the body through the water will take care of this handicap later.

    Bend forward at the waist, take a quick breath, go into a tuck, drawing the knees to the chest, chin to knees, and clasp arms around the legs. To recover footing, simply straighten the legs and stand up.

Prone Glide and Recovery—Glide back to the side of the pool; one foot flat against the side wall 10 to 12 inches from the bottom; arms and hands on top of the water. Inhale, submerge face, and give a gentle shove away from the bank with the raised foot. The body is in a straight line from the outstretch arms to toes. When the forward glide is spent, tuck legs, as sitting down in a chair, press hands down through water toward the knees, and stand.

Back Glide and Recovery—Face side of pool and place both hands in the gutter. Put one foot against the side of the pool, inhale, and shove into glide. As the forward motion is spent, bend knees, drop arms palms up, and vigorously pull arms in an arc toward the surface; lower feet and stand.

Following are some methods of staying afloat with minimum effort:

Horizontal Float—Divide the class into couples. Number ones face the side of the pool in waist-deep water; number twos stand directly behind them. Number ones assume a semi-sitting position with knees bent and hands in gutter. They inhale and lie back on the water by gradually straightening the legs and extending the arms obliquely. Number twos assist, if needed, by placing the fingertips or the palm of the hand in the small of the back or on the back of the head.

Finning—Check and see how many children have seen fish swim and then have them imitate the motions of the pectoral fins with the right hand, the left hand, and both hands. This should be done first above the water and then on the surface to get the feel of the water resistance. Lower the arms to sides, flex wrists, and push the water toward the feet. Now, get in the horizontal float position and repeat this motion. Better propulsion is obtained if the arms are kept fairly close to the sides.

Sculling—Have the learners imagine that the water is sand. With the arms extended and resting on top of the water, pull hands toward each other until the thumbs touch. There is a mound of sand between the hands. Turn the thumbs down and spread the sand out, pushing to the side. Repeat these motions until they become easy and rhythmic. The process of pull-in and push-out resembles that of frosting a cake, only it is done with both hands. Make a figure eight in the water with both hands. Lie back in float position and repeat motions.

Treading—Hold to the gutter with one hand and keep body erect and at right angles to the side of the pool; use free hand in finning or sculling motion and at the same time employ galloping, bicycling, or scissor action of the feet and legs. As skill progresses, release hand from gutter and employ both hands instead of one.

Strokes

ELEMENTARY BACKSTROKE. *Arms:* Start from back float to glide position, arms along side. Drop elbows toward bottom of pool, slide hands along sides of the legs and body until hands reach the chest, turn fingers outward; extend arms to full length, grasping water with the palms of both hands and press parallel with the water until hands have reached the sides of the body. *Legs:* Simultaneous with the action of the arms, spread knees slightly and, as arms are extended, step with feet into a "V" position. Catch the water with the soles of the feet, squeeze legs together to back glide position. Arms and legs work in unison followed by a glide.

Many handicapped persons find swimming on their backs to be the most fun and easiest of all swimming activities. The paraplegic who cannot move his legs can do this stroke by using only his arms; those lacking arm strength can learn to do it by using only their legs, for sculling and finning motions can be substitutes for total arm movements.

Strapping a float or flutter board between the legs will restrict their movements and develop increased arm strength for those needing to develop power in this part of the body.

SIDE STROKE. Shove off in lying position on either side with arm on underneath side fully extended above head and the other arm lying along side of the body, legs together and extended. Grasp the water with the underneath hand and press backward and downward at a 45-degree angle to a point directly in front of the chin. The side arm comes forward in rhythm with the lead arm to retrieve the water and is pushed toward feet and side. The leg action is coordinated with the movement of the side arm. Pull knees up slightly, step forward with the top leg, reach backward with the other leg to a wide arc, squeeze legs together, and glide.

This stroke is expecially beneficial for those having use of only one arm or leg. Those whose legs have both been amputated should learn to do this stroke in a partial prone position.

BREAST STROKE. The breast stroke can be taught with the face above water or with rhythmic breathing, submerging face during the glide. Shove off in a prone glide position. Grasp the water with the palms of the hands, press backward and downward until hands are parallel with the shoulders, pull elbows to sides of body, palms down, fingers pointing forward. Extend arms to starting position. As the arms are pressed backward and downward, drop knees. The outer edges of the feet are turned upward, toes outward. Push with the soles of the feet in an arc, outward and backward until the legs meet. Arms are extended as the leg action is completed, followed by a glide. Errors in timing may be avoided by allowing the learner to do only one complete stroke at a time until a perfect pattern has been set.

This stroke is often more easily learned by the mentally retarded than by other students. Blind people learning it should have both dry land and in-the-water practice, using first the arm movements as guided by the hands of a helper, then doing only the leg motions, and finally (with the aid of two helpers, one to pattern the arms and the other the feet) doing the stroke correctly in the water.

THE FRONT CRAWL. The crawl can and should be taught from the beginning of swimming instruction. The modified stroke with the head out of the water and a rapid and sporadic arm and leg action has been called the "human stroke" by the American Red Cross and the "dog paddle" by others. This stroke is gradually molded into the true crawl as the mental set and muscular coordination matures to the point where the learner can cope with the highly coordinated combination of leg thrash, arm cycle, and rhythmic breathing. *Legs:* The leg action is the same as that used in the back crawl except that the downward pressure with the instep and the upward lift with the sole of the foot is equal. *Arms:* Lift the elbow, using the shoulder muscles and letting forearm and hand hang relaxed; lead forward with the elbow and extend arm fully; cup hand and pull water to hip. Alternate right and left arms.

This stroke is difficult for many to learn, yet all who do so enjoy it the most. Movements of the arms or legs should be lessened for those whose joints are weak or stiff.

A "fun time" of 5 to 10 minutes is the perfect ending for a learning period in the water. The student leaves the pool relaxed and with a sustained enthusiasm that carries over to the next teaching period. The games and races utilize the simplest to the more advanced skills and give impetus to desire to master these skills in the formal teaching period.

It is recommended that for children 6 to 9, this period be used purely for play. Later, when the competitive spirit begins to run high, teams may be selected for a semester and a running score kept on the contests. Relays may be used instead of races when the groups are large.

Shallow-Water Activities

See how many can hold their breath and sit on the bottom of the pool.

See how many can submerge, holding their breath, and count their fingers.

Blow small sailboats, balloons, or ping-pong balls across the pool.

Poison Tag: "It" tries to tag a player who is safe while floating, finning, or sculling.

Corks: Throw in 10 corks. See who can collect the most.

Retrieving: Throw smooth rocks, lead washers, pucks and tin plates into the pool. See who can collect the most objects in a prescribed time.

Water Dodgeball: This promotes a feeling of security in the water.

Tunnel Ball: Divide into teams and pass ball between the legs.

Can You Do It?: Divide into two groups, selecting a leader for each group. The leader of one group performs a stunt. If the opposing team cannot do it, he receives a point for his team. Teams alternate in performing stunts.

Drop the Puck: The players form a circle and "It" drops the puck behind another player, who must retrieve it and try to catch "It" before he returns to the vacant place.

Life Line: Divide into teams. One member takes a position on the opposite side of the pool. At the whistle, each student drops into the pool and advances, joining hands with the others. Upon reaching the lone player, they try to get him back to their starting point quickly. This is not only a game but a device for rescuing weak swimmers who have stepped over their depth.

Leap Frog: Line up teams as for the game on land. The No. 1 player who returns to the head of the line first wins the game for his team.

Races using finning, sculling, and elementary strokes. In these, distance should be limited to proficiency of swimmers.

Underwater Race: 10 to 20 feet

Bobbing Race: Use bobbing technique and lunge body forward as it shoots to surface.

Flutterboard Relay: Use flutterboard with the flutter or whip kick. This may also be used for advanced swimmers.

Deep-Water Activities

The game program, for swimmers who can handle themselves in deep water, can be as varied and as interesting as the ingenuity of the instructor. Many land games and team games can be adapted to use in the water. Hula hoops or old basketball hoops serve as goals; wooden beads float on ropes and describe the playing area; old volleyball nets may be stretched across the pool with short standards and improvised vises attached to the gutters.

Water Baseball: Use bat and plastic ball. The diamond may be limited to shallow water, deep water, or both. Use regulation baseball rules.

Water Volleyball: Use water polo ball. Anchor net 3 feet above water. Mark limits with floating beads. Follow regulation volleyball rules.

Water Basketball: Place goals on sides of pool, if width permits. Play as in land basketball.

Modified Water Polo: Because water polo requires a great deal of stamina, its use must be limited to the more capable children. The play area should also be limited. The goals of two 3-foot uprights and crossbar 10 feet wide may be made of half-inch galvanized pipe and anchored to the sides and gutters. The goal should clear the water by 3 feet. Two teams of 7 to 10 line up in front of their respective goals.

Testing

The tests that follow have been made simpler and graded down for young children and, although they require the same skill, the reduced distances involved demand less stamina. The suggested names for the tests could be changed to fit the need; the last test could be divided into two if it is too difficult for the group. Small fish made of felt, in school colors, with the size increasing for graded tests could be stitched on bathing suits or trunks. Certain days should be set aside for testing and a routine followed; a child should be given credit for any completed skill whether it is in sequence or not.

Fingerling Test

1. *Breath-holding*—Take deep breath, submerge, and pick up four objects in a 12-inch radius.
2. *Bobbing*—Executed 10 times in a deliberate manner. Should not finish gasping for breath.
3. *Prone Float*—Horizontal position if possible. If feet sink to bottom, points should be given on the relaxation of the swimmer.
4. *Prone Glide and Recovery*—Body should plane through water and after the glide is spent, recovery should be unhurried.
5. *Back Glide and Recovery*—Same as front, except head raised slightly.
6. *Back Float*—Horizontal; semi-horizontal; knees bent or vertical position acceptable.
7. *Finning*—Hands close to sides.
8. *Sculling*—Described figure eight. Definite propulsion through water.
9. *Crawl*—Dog Paddle; arms may be under water or out. Rhythmic breathing not required. Distance only requirement.
10. *Elementary Back*—Fair amount of form expected because coordination is simple.
11. *Dives and Jumps* (shoulder-depth water)—Level off and swim 10 feet.

Keeper Test

1. *Elementary Back*—Good form required.
2. *Tread Water*—Hands allowed.
3. *Side Stroke*—Fair form; grade 3 (on swimming stroke sheet) should be a passing grade.
4. *Underwater Swim*—Two body lengths.
5. *Jump into Deep Water*—Level off and swim to bank of shallow water.
6. *Standing Front Dive*—Do not grade for form. Head-first entry only requirement.
7. *Sculling*—Good form and relaxed.
8. *Crawl*—Arms should clear water and fair degree of coordination expected in arms, legs, and rhythmic breathing. 3 passing grade.
9. *Surface Dive*—Toes should go under water without swimming assist.
10. *Turn Over*—Change from back to side or front and continue to swim for several feet.
11. *Kick Glide*—Flutter kick for 20 feet on back or front without use of hands or arms.
12. *Three-Minute Swim*—Use any stroke and sculling or finning.

Fish Test

All strokes should be done in good form. If a board is available, the front dive should be done from it, otherwise from the bank.

SUGGESTED READINGS

American Association for Health, *Football Skills Test Manual* (Boys); *Basketball Skills Test Manual* (Boys) (Girls); *Softball Skills Test Manual* (Boys) (Girls). Washington, D.C.: AAHPER, 1966.

———, *Official Aquatic Guide*. Washington, D.C.: AAHPER, 1975.

———, *Practical Guide for Teaching the Mentally Retarded to Swim; An Annotated Bibliography: Swimming For The Handicapped,* Washington, D.C.: AAHPER, 1969.

———, Division of Girls' and Women's Sports:

Guides: *Aquatics,* 1965–67; *Archery, Riding,* 1966–68; *Bowling, Fencing, Golf,* 1964–66; *Field Hockey, Lacrosse,* 1966–68; *Gymnastics,* 1965; *Outing Activities and Winter Sports,* 1965–67; *Soccer, Speedball,* 1966–68; *Softball,* 1966–68; *Tennis, Badminton,* 1966–68; *Track and Field,* 1966–68; *Volleyball,* 1965–67. (These guides contain official rules for players and officials, and selected articles. All guides except the basketball guide are published biannually.)

Reprint Series: *Selected Aquatics Articles,* 1964; *Selected Basketball Articles,* 1964; *Selected Field Hockey-Lacrosse Articles,* 1963; *Selected Soccer-Speedball Articles,* 1963; *Selected Softball Articles,* 1962; *Selected Tennis-Badminton Articles,* 1963; *Selected Volleyball Articles,* 1960.

Technique Charts: *Aquatics-Swimming and Diving* (18 charts); *Badminton* (12 charts); *Basketball* (12 charts); *Bowling*—Ten-Pin (9 charts, boys and girls); *Softball* (11 charts); *Speedball* (8 charts); *Tennis* (12 charts); *Volleyball* (11 charts).

American Red Cross, *Swimming and Diving*, rev. ed. Washington, D.C.: American Red Cross, 1975.

————, *Rescue and Water Safety* (Lifesaving). Washington, D.C.: American Red Cross, 1975.

ANDERSON, WILLIAM, *Teaching the Physically Handicapped to Swim*. New York: Translantic Arts, 1968.

ARMBRUSTER, D. A., R. H. ALLEN, and H. S. BILLINGSLEY, *Swimming and Diving*, 4th ed. St. Louis: C. V. Mosby, 1963.

BELLISIMO, LOU, *The Bowlers Manual*, 2nd ed. Englewood Cliffs, N.J.: Prentice-Hall, 1969.

BLAKE, WILLIAM, *Lead-up Games to Team Sports*. Englewood Cliffs, N.J.: Prentice-Hall, 1964.

GABRIELSEN, M. A., BETTY SPEARS, and B. W. GABRIELSEN, *Aquatics Handbook*. Englewood Cliffs, N.J.: Prentice-Hall, 1960.

KAUFFMAN, CAROLYN, *How to Teach Children to Swim*. New York: G. P. Putnam's Sons, 1960.

KING, ELEANOR, ed., *How We Do It Game Book*, 3rd ed. Washington, D.C.: AAHPER, 1964.

MIDTLYNG, JOANNA, *Swimming*. Philadelphia: W. B. Saunders, 1974.

The Saunders Physical Activities Series. Philadelphia: W. B. Saunders, 1970–1976.

Archery—Lorraine Pszczola
Bowling—Carol Shunk
Golf—Billye Anne Cheatum
Gymnastics for Girls and Women—Betty Roys
Jogging for Fitness and Weight Control—Frederick Roby and Russell Davis
Power Volleyball—Thomas Slaymaker and Virginia Brown
Soccer—C. Ian Bailey and Francis Teller
Tennis—Robert Gensemer
Track and Field Activities for Girls and Women—Virginia Parker and Robert Kennedy
Tumbling for Men and Women—Vannie Edwards

SHAFFER, J. LAVERE, "An Aiming Device for Teaching Archery to the Blind," *D.G.W.S. Archery Guide* (1966–1968), p. 28.

SMITH, HOPE, *Water Games*. New York: Ronald Press, 1962.

VANNIER, MARYHELEN, and HALLY BETH POINDEXTER, *Individual and Team Sports for Girls and Women*, 3rd ed. Philadelphia: W. B. Saunders, 1976.

VARNER, MARGARET, *Badminton*. Dubuque, Iowa: Brown, 1966.

14

Rhythms,
Movement Exploration,
and Dance

Rhythms, movement exploration and folk, social, and modern dance can provide wholesome, satisfying recreation for many of the handicapped as well as the normal. Festivals, recitals, shows, and other types of public demonstration will add richness and variety to the program.

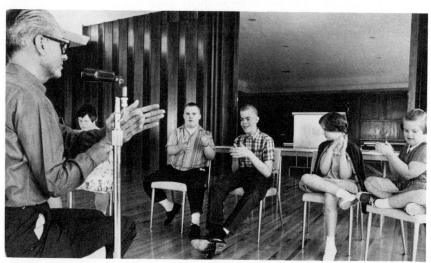

The physical educator should be able to teach a wide variety of activities. Here, rhythm is being taught. Courtesy of the AAHPER.

The ideal facility for learning movements, rhythms, and dances is a polished hardwood floor big enough to accommodate twenty or more couples. However, any smooth surface will do, even an asphalt tennis court, a multipurpose concrete surface, or a school corridor. Street dances held in roped-off areas are recommended for large numbers and adding variety to the program.

Music is, of course, vital in teaching these activities. A public address system is best if it has two speakers, a turntable or phonograph which plays 78, 33⅓, and 45 r.p.m. records and has adjustable speed control, a microphone, and an amplifier. The use of a live band is ideal for dances. However, because many excellent folk, social, and square dance records with directions are available, they are handy for teaching. All such records should be indexed, labeled, and stored in albums or metal carrying cases.

BASIC RHYTHMS

Children and the older mentally retarded delight in taking part in a rhythm band. Although drums, tambourines, shakers, and other instruments can be purchased from music firms, the participants in this program will more enjoy making and playing their own homemade musical instruments. The leader should ever be on the lookout for discarded materials from which useful articles can be made. Below are some suggested instruments:

1. Drums can be made from pieces of inner tube stretched over cans of varying sizes. Beaters can be made from heavy sticks padded and covered with cloth.
2. Tambourines can be made from two paper plates sewed front to front with yarn. Tie tiny bells on metal discs around the edges. Tin pie plates can be pasted or nailed together with tiny rocks or rice inside to make a sound.
3. Shakers and rattles can be made by partly filling cans with rice, popcorn, or rocks. Cut a hole in one end, insert a stick handle, and paint in a bright color.
4. Sand blocks can be made from two wooden blocks, chalkboard size, covered with emery paper to make a scratching noise when rubbed together.
5. Wooden sticks to hit together can be made from dowels or a broom handle cut 6 inches or longer.
6. Bottles and glasses set in a row, each with varying amounts of different colored water, will make melodic sounds when tapped with a metal spoon.
7. A uke box can be made from a box. Notches are cut on each end and rubber bands are stretched into each one at each end.
8. A clapper can be made by loosely nailing one or two roofing discs (available from any hardware store) on top of each other on thin flat boards. These are struck into the palm of one hand.

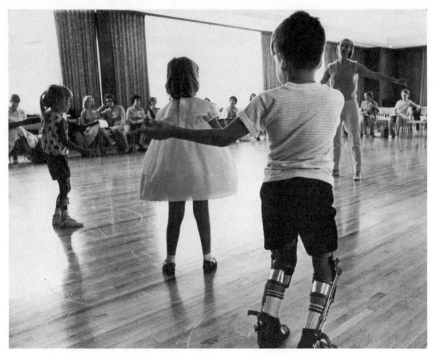
Exercising to music is much more fun! Courtesy of the AAHPER.

9. Brightly colored ribbons on which small bells are sewed can be made to wear or shake.
10. A washboard rubbed by a spoon makes a good instrument.

For a rhythm band to be the most fun, peppy records should provide the melody and give the players the emphasis for each beat. Marching, skipping, and hopping can be added as accompaniments to the sounds. If the group is large and the instruments few, half of the class can play for the others as they perform, and vice versa.

MOVEMENT EXPLORATION

Children love to explore, to find how many ways they can move in space, and see how fast or slowly they can do small or large movements. The teacher poses problems such as "How many ways can you jump up and down?" or "Who can run the fastest, the slowest, and the most quiet?" etc.

Movement exploration can best be done in a gymnasium or an empty classroom. Many kinds of equipment can be used. A large variety will add interest to the program. Suggestions are:

Many 2 × 4 boards for jumping and balancing	Teeter-totters
Ropes of varying lengths	Boxes of all sizes and shapes
Broomsticks, wands	1 beanbag for every child
Jungle gyms, bars	Climbing steps and ladders
Fold-up or long mats	Blocks and balls of varying sizes
	Cargo nets

252

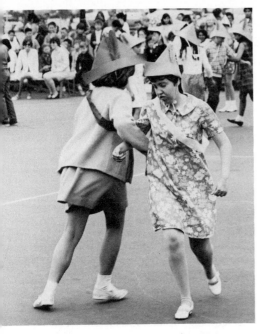

Children learn as much from each other as they do from adults. Courtesy of the Los Angeles Public Schools.

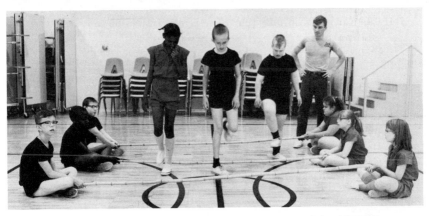

Parallel poles are helpful in learning how to balance. Courtesy of the AAHPER.

Benches	Parachutes
Low turning bars	Telephone poles or large tree
Stilts and tin can walkers	trunks for climbing
Single and long jumpropes	Balance boards
Trampolines	Hula hoops

Suggested Locomotor Activities

Walking

1. How many tiny or giant steps does it take you to cross this room?
2. Can you change your direction (Level? Speed?) and still keep walking?
3. Can you express joy when walking? Sorrow? Anger?

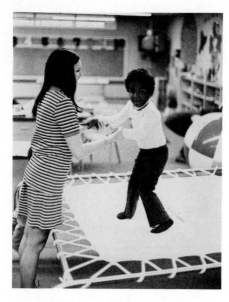

The trampoline can be used to explore body movements in the air and upon landing. Courtesy of the Richardson, Texas Public Schools.

4. Can you walk on only your toes? Heels? Insides of your feet? Outside?
5. Discover how many ways you can walk.

Running

1. Run and stop fast when you hear the whistle.
2. Who can run in the greatest number of different ways?
3. Can you combine a run with any other kind of movement, such as a jump?
4. If you can run forward, how many other ways can you run?
5. Can you run using your arms in a way other than swinging them forward and backward?

Hopping

1. Hop as fast as you can on one foot.
2. Jump as lightly as you can on both feet.
3. Combine a hop with another movement.
4. Hop in a circle. See how many other ways you can hop.
5. Jump as high as you can five times; then lower your body every time you hop for five more times. Who can hop lowest to the floor?

Sliding

1. See how many ways you can slide other than forward.
2. Combine a slide with any other kind of movement.
3. Slide around in a circle with a partner.
4. Slide in a big circle with two others. Can you find a way to go in and out of a circle while sliding?
5. Can you slide face to face then back to back with a partner?

Skipping

1. Skip forward, skip in a big circle, then on a diagonal.
2. Can you skip holding hands with a partner?
3. How many others can skip with you holding hands?
4. How fast can you skip? How slowly?
5. Can you change from a skip to a slide or a gallop?

Jumping

1. How many times can you jump up and down on one foot? On both feet?
2. Can you jump going around in a circle? In a square? Forward? Backward?
3. Who can jump first on one foot and then on the other for the longest time?
4. Can you jump from the top of this box or table to the mat below?
5. Can you jump, run, jump, skip?

General Locomotor Activities

1. Choose a corner in this room. Run to it fast when I say "go!" Now do it very slowly.
2. Bend as far as you can forward, backward, and to the side as you walk forward.
3. Make yourself squat as low to the floor as you can. Stretch high as near to the ceiling as you can.
4. Raise your right arm and left leg, then your left arm and right leg while marching in place. Now march around the room.
5. As you run forward, change from being a tall giant to a tiny mouse, but keep moving.

Equipment

Turning Bar

1. Can you make a circle over this bar?
2. Who can chin himself on the bar?
3. Can you circle the bar using just one leg?
4. Who can "skin the cat" using this bar?
5. Can you reach behind you and by grasping the bar make a circle over it with your body?

The Climbing Ladder

1. See how fast you can go up and down the ladder.
2. Can you climb up the ladder without using your feet?
3. Can you weave in and out of the rungs to go up and come down the ladder?
4. Can you skip any rungs while climbing it?
5. What else can you do using this ladder?

The Stairs

1. Who can go up and down the stairs without holding onto a railing?
2. Can you go up and down them by hopping on two feet? One foot?
3. Can you go up and down backward? Jump up and down them facing sideward?
4. Can you walk up and down them balancing yourself by your hands?
5. Can you go up and down by moving over one, two, or more steps?

Sawed-Off Broomsticks or Wands

1. Can you balance the stick in the palm of your hand? On two fingers, then on one finger?
2. Can you throw it up into the air, spin around, and catch it before it hits the floor?
3. Can you play pitch and catch with it with a partner, using the same hand you catch it with to throw it?
4. Can you balance the stick while kneeling on one knee? Both knees? While slowly lying down and getting back up?
5. Can you twirl the stick while pretending to be a drum majorette?

Tires

1. See how fast you can roll the tire.
2. See if you can roll it in a circle. In a straight line. Backward.
3. Jump in and out of it, moving around in a circle if the tire is flat on the floor.
4. Can you crawl through it when someone holds it up?
5. Can you throw a volleyball through it? A baseball?

DANCE

Social dance is an especially good activity for the handicapped, for it can provide them with opportunities to have some physical contact with others, including the normal. Just touching another human being can be, in itself, a therapeutic experience. Moving in rhythm to a catchy tune is fun, and can add a spot of brightness to what otherwise for some is a drab life. The mentally retarded especially enjoy this type of activity. Wheelchair square dance is a favorite among the orthopedically handicapped.

Dance activities should range all the way from simple singing games for children to more complicated folk, square, and social dance patterns for adults. Creative movement activities are especially recommended for those emotionally disturbed or mentally ill. Dance activities are also popular among the deaf who, although unable to hear the music, can respond to the rhythm it makes through floor vibrations.

For some groups complicated dances should not be included in the program. For still others it is best to pair them off so that disabilities complement each other, thus a blind boy can be taught to social dance well with a sighted deaf girl. It is also wise to have a "highlight" program event periodically, such as a valentine dance party.

Dance exhibition groups who go from one community center, school, or church to another to "show" what they can do to those with similar handicaps, or to those who are classified as normal, can bring joy to the performers, a sense of pride to the parents of the dancers, and a greater understanding and insight to all watchers who believe that the handicapped "just can't do things as well as their normal peers."

Ballroom Dance

There are many kinds of ballroom dances that can be taught. Some are fast and energetic; some are slow, gliding, and relaxed. After the students have learned to play a variety of simple instruments, they will be ready to learn to move their bodies to music in structured dance forms such as the waltz, the samba, the rumba, and even some of the contemporary "rock" forms. This will depend largely on their *physical* capabilities, for even slow learners can find enjoyment and a certain degree of mastery in dancing. And it isn't necessary to have all of one's physical capacities intact to dance—even people in wheelchairs can move to specific forms and rhythms in structured dance movements. Body movement to music and rhythm is extremely enjoyable for most people; and it promotes physical, emotional, and social well-being with its relaxed atmosphere.

THE FOX-TROT

Fox-trot music may be fast, medium, or slow. The medium or medium-slow dance is easiest to learn· and the most popular. Music for the fox-trot is written in 4/4 time (four beats to each measure); however, four steps are not taken during each measure. The dance is done in this step pattern:

Slow	2 counts
Slow	2 counts
Quick	1 count
Quick	1 count

Each complete step requires six counts or beats—the equivalent of one and one-half measures. The words *slow* (S) and *quick* (Q) are especially descriptive of the step patterns.

The fox-trot is characterized by its long, smooth, gliding steps. The rhythm pattern is

$$\frac{1}{S} \quad 2 \quad \frac{3}{S} \quad 4 \qquad \frac{1}{Q} \quad 2 \quad \frac{3}{Q} \quad \frac{4}{S} \qquad \frac{1}{S} \quad 2 \quad \frac{3}{Q} \quad \frac{4}{Q}$$

Groups can discover the accented first and third beats of each measure by clapping to fox-trot music.

Arrange the group into a counterclockwise circle with the men moving forward and women backward. Call the slow, slow, quick, quick pattern and let the dancers follow. Practice this step in closed position. Introduce new steps as the group progresses. Demonstrate and practice several routines and encourage all to make up their own.

Steps

Basic Step

S   Step forward left
S   Step forward right
Q   Step sideways left
Q   Close right, transfer weight to right
Repeat beginning left again.

(This step may be referred to as an "L" step to help the dancers remember the pattern.)

Walking Step

S   Step forward left
S   Step forward right
S   Step forward left
S   Step forward right

Side Close Step

Q   Step sideways left
Q   Close right to left, transfer weight
S   Step sideways left

(The right foot is closed to the left during the "slow" count, but weight is not transferred.)

To progress forward using Side Close step:

Q   Step sideways left
Q   Close right to left
S   Step forward left

(The steps and the transfer of weight in this step are the same as those of the basic quarter-turns and half-turns.)

Dip

S   Step left backward
S   Step forward right, recovering the regular closed position
Q   To add "side close," step sideways left
Q   Close right to left

(The man should step backward with a medium-sized step to insure smooth, continuous movement. The man's left knee is turned slightly out to allow his partner to bend her right knee as she steps forward.)

Forward, Open Position

S   Step sideways left
S   Cross right foot in front of left, step right (left foot should "brush" by right to be in place for next step)

Q Step sideways left
Q Close right, transferring weight
(This step may be varied by a "turn-under": As the man steps sideways left, he turns the lady under her right arm. The lady pivots as she steps so that she completes a turn in time to take the second "quick" step, in regular closed position.)

Turns

Quarter-Turn

S Step sideways left
Q Close right to left, transfer weight
S Step forward left, turning toe out, pivot $\frac{1}{4}$ turn
Q Step sideways right
Q Close left to right
S Step back to right, turning toe in, pivot $\frac{1}{4}$ turn
Repeat this pattern to return to original position.

Half-Turn Right

S Step forward left
S Step forward right turning toe out, pivot $\frac{1}{4}$ turn
Q Step side left
Q Close right to left
S Turn shoulders to the right, step back left, pivot $\frac{1}{4}$ turn
Q Step sideways right
Q Close left to right
S Step forward right

Half-Turn Left

S Step forward left, toe out
Q Step sideways right
Q Close left to right
S Step back right, toe in
Q Step sideways left
Q Close right to left
S Step forward left

Combinations

Two-Step

Q Step left
Q Close right
S Step left
S Step right
S Step left
Repeat pattern, beginning right.

Dance-Walk with Side Close

Four dance-walk steps, beginning left:
S Step left
S Step right

Q   Step sideways left
Q   Close right to left
Repeat routine.

Dance-Walk, Side Close with Open Position

S   Step left
S   Step right
Q   Step sideways left
Q   Close right to left
Open position.
S   Step forward left
S   Step forward right
Return to closed position.
Q   Step side left
Q   Close right to left

Dance-Walk with Turn-Under

S   Step 4 walking steps
Open position.
S   Step left
S   Step right across or forward
Q   Step left, turning lady under
Q   Step right, returning to closed position

THE WALTZ

Begin with clapping the rhythm, accenting the first beat of each measure. The words "step, step, close" describe the waltz pattern much better than "quick, quick, slow." The box waltz is the easiest for beginners to learn.

Music for the American waltz is in medium slow tempo. Fast waltz tempo has its own special step, the Viennese Waltz. Most dance groups will enjoy learning how to do this as a climax to a class.

Steps

Box Waltz

Counts:
1   Step forward left
2   Step side right, "brush" by left making an angle
3   Close left to right, transfer weight
1   Step back right
2   Step side left
3   Close right to left, transfer weight
Repeat entire pattern.

Half-Squares to Progress Forward

Counts:
1   Step forward left
2   Step side right

3   Close left to right, transfer weight
1   Step forward right
2   Step side left
3   Close right to left

Hesitation Waltz (for variation of pattern)

Counts:
1   Step forward left
2   Swing right forward
3   Touch right toe forward past left, leg extended
1   Step backward right
2   Swing left backward
3   Touch left toe to floor past right, leg extended

(Actually, the dancers step only on the first beat of each measure.)

Left Turn

Counts:
1   Step forward and to the side left, toe turned out
2   Step side right
3   Close left to right
1   (4) Step backward right, toe turned in
2   (5) Step side left
3   (6) Close right to left
Repeat counts 1 through 6 to complete turn.

Right Turn

Counts:
1   Step forward and to the side right, toe turned out
2   Step side left
3   Close right to left
1   (4) Step backward left, toe turned in
2   (5) Step side right
3   (6) Close left to right
Repeat counts 1 through 6 to complete turn.

THE TANGO

Tango music is in 2/4 time with a special accent in rhythm that tells the dancer when to step and when to pause. First, play several tangos to let the group listen. Discuss the accents and the style of the music. Next, have them clap out the rhythm.

The basic step is the dance walk with a slight variation. The dancer bends his knee as he steps and lifts his foot up off the floor to carry out the characteristic tango style. The steps are smooth, deliberate, and long.

Again the words *slow* and *quick* are valuable. The basic pattern of the dance is slow, slow, quick, quick, slow; the steps are forward, forward, forward, side, draw. In the draw, one foot closes to the other foot, but no weight is transferred to the closing foot. After the dancers have listened to music and have repeated slow, slow, quick, quick, slow several

times, have them step in time with the words, then progress to the basic
step—the step, side draw. Variations are again introduced as soon as the
group has practiced the first step in closed social dance position.

Steps

Promenade

    S   Step forward left
    S   Step forward right
    S   Step forward left
    Q   Step forward right
    S   Step forward left
    Repeat, beginning on right.

Side Close

    S   Step forward left
    Q   Step forward right
    Q   Step sideways left (short step)
    S   Close right to left, transfer weight

Side Draw

    S   Step forward left
    S   Step forward right
    Q   Step forward left
    Q   Step sideways right
    S   Draw left to right, weight remains on right

Pivot Turn Left

    Open Position
    S   Step forward left (lady right)
    S   Step across right, lady steps left then pivots on left into closed position
    Q   Step forward left (small step)
    Q   Step sideways right
    S   Draw left to right

Pivot Turn Right (directions to man)

    Open position as in left turn
    S   Step forward left
    S   Step forward right, pivot on right foot into closed position
    Q   Step backward left
    Q   Step sideways right
    S   Draw left to right

Step-Out with Sweep Pivot (directions to man)

    Open position
    S   Step forward left
    S   Step forward right, swing left leg in a circle, cross over right
    Q   Closed position, step left
    Q   Step side right
    S   Draw left to right

The Corte

    Q Step forward left
    Q Step back in place right
    S Dip backward left
    S Recover
    Q Step forward right
    Q Step side left
    S Draw right to left

THE RUMBA

The rumba has the 4/4 time and the key words "quick, quick, slow" in common with the fox-trot. However, special features of the rumba definitely distinguish it from the smooth, even fox-trot, so the dancer cannot fox-trot a little faster and call his dance a rumba.

To do this Cuban dance, the upper part of the body moves only slightly while hip and knee action create a continuous, flowing movement from the waist down. Half-size steps are taken with the foot flat on the floor.

The step and the transfer of weight occur at different times. When one foot is moved, no weight is shifted until the other foot is in position to step. Always, one knee is bent in taking a step; the other is straight, holding the body weight. This delayed action causes the hips to move. The closed position is used with one variation. The man's left arm and the lady's right are bent at the elbow with their hands held at eye level.

Steps

Practice Pattern (two rumba steps)

Begin with feet together.
Counts:
1 Shift weight to right foot; step left, foot flat on floor, knee bent, no weight
2 Straighten left knee, take weight; close right to left, right knee bent, no weight
3 Straighten right knee, take weight; relax left knee, step forward
4 Hold

Rumba Box or Square

    Q Step sideways left
    Q Close right to left
    S Step forward left
    Q Step right sideways
    Q Close left to right
    S Step backward right

The Running Step

    Q Step forward left; hips move to right
    Q Step forward right; hips move to left

S   Step forward left; hips move to right

(This last step and hip swing should be done slowly so that the movement will take two full beats, beats 3 and 4.)

The Turn (lady)

Man leads lady into open position. He raises his left arm and turns lady to her right in a clockwise circle under his left arm.

Man continues to dance the rumba square in place, lady dances the running step.

The Circle Turn (lady)

Man retains lady's right hand in his left. Partners rumba away from each other until arms are straightened.

Man leads the lady to his right. When his hands are near his right side, he takes the lady's right hand in his right hand and transfers it to his left again behind his back.

As the lady returns to face her partner he raises his left hand and arm and returns to closed position.

THE SAMBA

The Samba is a delightful Brazilian dance in which the dancer rocks to a rhythm with an accented beat. As soon as a person learns the basic step, he can begin creating his own routines.

Samba music is written in 4/4 time, but actually the dance steps indicate that the time is quick, quick, slow, with the first quick step more heavily accented than the second. The characteristic movement of the dance is an up-and-down bounce, created by bending and straightening the knees on every step while the dancer sways or bends the body from the knees up in the opposite direction to the way the feet move.

Steps

Practice Pattern for the Basic Step

Q   Step forward left, knee bent
Q   Step forward right, closing right parallel to left foot; transfer weight, straighten both knees
S   Step left in place, both knees bent
Q   Step back right, knee bent slightly
Q   Step back left, close to right, knees bent
S   Step in place right, knees bent

As the dancer steps forward left, the upper part of his body sways backward, bending from the knees. Then the body sways forward as the dancer steps backward. This basic step is done in closed position. Two popular variations are the butterfly break and the marcha or shuffle step. Routines should be done in fours or multiples of four. The lead indications should be given during the last steps in a series of four.

The Butterfly Break—Reverse Open (couples face man's right, lady's left)

Q Step side left
Q Place right toe directly behind left heel and rock weight to toe
S   Step in place left; transfer weight; return weight to left

The Butterfly Break—Open Position

Q Step side right
Q Place left toe behind right heel and rock weight to toe
S   Step in place right, returning weight to right

(In this break, the dancers bend from the waist in the direction in which they step. Also, they should look over their shoulders toward the floor to lend style to their dance.)

The Marcha or Shuffle—Open or Conversation Position

S   Step forward left, knees bent
S   Straighten left knee quickly; shift weight momentarily to right foot; pull left foot slightly backward and in the same motion, bend left knee, taking all weight on left

Square Dance

Square dancing is well-established as a recreational activity. Even the drawback of providing a caller has been eliminated by recordings both of singing and patter calls that come complete with dance music and instructions.

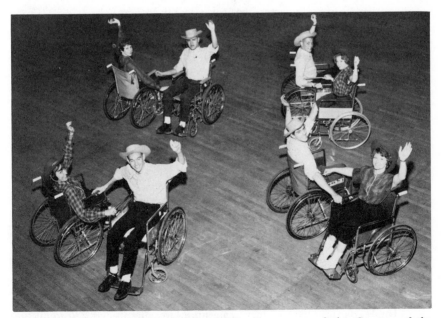

Wheelchair square dancing is a favorite activity of many paraplegics. Courtesy of the AAHPER.

Few people learn to square dance without good leadership; here again the recreation director must take on the role of teacher. Disabled people may be interested and enthusiastic, but without skillful teaching they will soon settle down to the "wallflower," observing role.

Square dancing can be very simple or extremely complicated. Following is a list of square dance terms teachers will need to know to teach this activity. These are provided to briefly indicate the level of skills needed for basic square dancing.

All Get Straight—Couples get in proper order (couple 4 on right of couple 3, etc.).

Allemande Left—Give left hand to corner and swing one time around.

Allemande Right—(Follows "allemande left.") Swing partner once around right hand.

Balance—Each partner steps two steps backward and bows, then takes two steps forward back to the original position.

Balance and Swing—Two steps backward; forward again to swing partner once around with a waist swing.

Bar—The position from which a dancer starts a figure.

Break—To release hands.

Break and Trail—Release hands, turn to the right, and move single file back to home position.

Center—The middle of the square formed by the dancers.

Circle Eight—All four couples join hands and move to the left.

Corner—The person across the "corner" of the square.

Corner Lady—The lady on the man's left.

Divide the Ring—One couple crosses the square to couple opposite them, passes between that pair. The lady turns to her right and the man to his left, and they move outside the square to return to their home position.

Do-Si-Do—Give your partner your left hand; swing him/her around. Give corner your right hand, and swing that person once around. Go back to partner, and promenade home. When the call "one more turn" is given, repeat the figure: partner, left; corner, right; partner left again; corner right again; then promenade home.

Dos-A-Dos—Partners face each other; advance, passing right shoulders. Step to the right without turning around, then move backward to starting position (facing partner).

Elbow Swing—Hook right elbows with the person you are to swing and swing once or once and a half around as the call directs.

Figure—The main part of the dance. A dance is identified by the name of its figure.

Forward and Back—Take four steps into the center and four steps back to place.

Grand Right and Left—Partners take right hands in handshake position, and pass right shoulders. They give the next person in the circle their left hands, and pass left shoulders, continuing weaving in and out around the circle until they meet at the opposite side of the square. The couples promenade home unless the call directs them to continue the grand right and left until they are back to home position. This call usually follows "allemande left."

Head Couples—The first and third couples.

Home Position—The first position of each couple in the square. The man always returns to this first position at the call "promenade home."

Honor Your Partner—Ladies curtsy to their partners; men bow.

Honor Your Corner—Ladies curtsy to their corners; each man bows to his corner lady.

Ladies Chain—Two couples face each other. Each lady moves toward the other; they join right hands and pass right shoulders. Then the lady gives her left hand to the opposite man; he turns her once around. The ladies again join right hands and pass through back to their partners who turn them around to original position.

Lead Out—Call for one couple to move in some particular direction.

On to the Next—Call for couple or man to advance to the next couple to the right.

Opposite—The person or couple directly across the set.

Promenade—Each man takes his partner in skater's position, and all the couples move counterclockwise around the circle. In this position, the partners stand side by side, lady on the man's right. The man takes his lady's left hand in his left hand, and her right hand in his right. His right arm is over her left arm.

Right Hands Across—Men join right hands and move clockwise. This call is also given to the ladies of the set.

Sashay—See *Dos-A-Dos*.

See-Saw—See *Dos-A-Dos*.

Set—See *Square*.

Side Couples—Second and fourth couples.

Square—Four couples in an arrangement that forms a square. Each couple makes one side of the square. The couple with their backs to the music is the number one or head couple. Couple two is on the right of couple one; three is opposite, and four is to the left of the head couple. The first couple begins each figure unless otherwise designated.

Swing

    Two-Step Swing—Partners take closed social dance position, then move to the left until their right sides are touching. The lady and the man both step forward on the left foot and continue moving in place, clockwise, by dancing a series of two-steps. Partners pull away from each other, making possible a "whirling" motion.

    Pivot Swing—Partners take position described above. The partners pivot around clockwise on their right feet, pulling away from the "center" of the pivot as in the two-step swing.

    Right- or Left-Hand Swing—The lady and man join right or left hands and swing around. Their arms are bent at the elbow; they extend their fingers up and catch hands at eye level. (This is in contrast to the handshake position.)

Two-Hand Swing—The couple joins both hands and swings around, facing one another.

Waist Swing—The man places his hands at the lady's waist; the lady rests her hands on the man's shoulders, and they swing to the right (clockwise).

Taw—Partner.

Twirl—The man holds the lady's right hand in his right hand; raises their right arms, and turns the lady under his right arm until she is in promenade position.

OPENING CALLS

Honor your corner, and the lady by your side,
Now all join hands and circle out wide.
Round and round and round you go,
And you break that ring with a do-si-do, and a little more do,
Chicken in the bread pan a'peckin' out dough.
Grab your partner and home you go.

All jump up and never come down. (Dancers yell as they jump.)
Swing your little girl 'round and 'round,
'Till the hollow of your foot makes a hole in the ground.
Promenade, boys, promenade.

Honor your partner, and the lady on your left.
All join hands and circle to the left.
Swing your corner like swingin' on a gate.
Right to your partner and right and left eight.
One foot up and the other one down.
Meet your partner as she comes down,
Swing her round and round,
And promenade home.

Honor your partner, honor your corner.
All join hands and circle eight.
And you circle eight and all get straight.
Allemande left with your left hand,
Right to your partner and right and left grand.
Meet ole Sal and meet ole Sue and
Meet that gal with a rundown shoe.
All promenade, boys, promenade.

All eight balance,
All eight swing, and promenade around the ring.
Promenade!

All join hands and circle eight.
Break and trail along that line,
Ladies in the lead and the gents behind.
Swing your partner and promenade home.

Note: These calls may be used also as mixers or fillers by omitting the call "Honor your partner."

ENDING CALLS

Honor your partner,
Honor your corner,
Wave to your opposite,
That's all.

Promenade, and I don't care.
Take her to that high-back chair.

Swing your partner,
Pat her on the head,
Take her out and feed her cornbread.

Swing your corner,
Swing your own,
And there you stand!

DO-SI-DO PATTER

Do-si-do, and a little more do,
Hurry up boys, can't be slow.
You'll never get to heaven if you don't do so.
One more change, and home you go.

Do-si-do, and a little more do,
Chicken in the bread pan scratchin' out gravel.
Grab your gal, and home you travel.

Do-si-do—partner left—
Corner right—
Back to your partner, and home you go.

Do-si-do, and a little more do,
Aces high and deuces low.
One more change, and on you go.

Do-si-do, and here we go,
With a little bit of heel, and a little bit of toe,
Meet your partner and home you go.

DANCES

Hot Time in the Old Town
    Music: Any recording of the song that is peppy.

All four girls, to the center of the ring.   Girls form center ring moving clock-
                                        wise.

All four boys, promenade around the ring.	Boys circle in opposite direction.
Pass your partner, the next one you will swing,	Boy swings his right hand girl.
There'll be a Hot Time in the Old Town Tonight.	
(Repeat three more times, until all boys are back to their original partners.)	Same as above.
All four boys, to the center of the ring.	Boys form center ring moving clockwise.
All four girls, promenade around the ring.	Girls circle in opposite direction.
Pass your partner, the next one you will swing,	Girl swings with next boy.
There'll be a Hot Time in the Old Town Tonight.	

(Repeat three more times, until all boys are with original partners. Use any ending call.)

Oh! Johnny

Music: The Tune "Oh! Johnny" or the recorded singing call.

All join hands and circle the ring.	Circle 8 left.
Stop where you are and give your partner a swing.	Waist swing your partner twice around.
Now swing the girl behind you.	Waist swing your corner lady.
Swing your own if you think you have time to.	Swing your partner again.
Allemande left on your corners all.	Swing once around your corner lady, and face your partner.
And dos-a-dos your own.	Sashay your partner, and turn to face your corner.
Then all promenade with that sweet corner maid,	Promenade your corner.
Singing, "Oh, Johnny, O, Johnny, Oh!"	Promenade home—and sing!

(Repeat three times until each man has his original partner.)

Sally Goodin (all couples dancing)

Music: "Sally Goodin."

Four men out, and swing Sally Goodin with your right hand.	Each man steps behind his partner, and moves to his right hand lady. He swings her once around with his right hand.
Now swing your taw.	Men return to partners and swing once around with left hand.
Swing that girl from Arkansas.	Man swings his corner lady with left hand swing, once around.
Now swing your taw.	Left hand swing with partner.

And don't forget to swing Grandmaw,

With a two-hand swing.
Back to your partner,

And everybody swing.

And promenade your corner around the ring.

Men move to the right in the center of the square to the opposite lady.
Swing opposite once around.
Men again circle to the right to return home.
Everyone swings with a waist swing. The man should swirl his partner around the set to the next position, so that she will be ready to promenade.
Promenade home.

(Repeat three times, until the ladies are at their original home position.)

Uptown and Downtown

Music: Any square dance recording of "Golden Slippers."

Beginning pattern.
First couple up center and away uptown.

Bring that other couple down.
Pick them up and let them fall.
Here you go all around the hall.
Lady go gee and gent go haw,

Right elbow swing as you did before,

Elbow swing as you go round,
And swing your corner lady.
Swing your corner lady, swing her round and round.
Now all promenade, go round the town, promenade around.
Tap your heel and save your toe,
Chicken in the breadpan scratching dough,
Places all and hear my call, ready, ready, here we go!

First couple, hands joined, walk to couple 3, bring them back to couple 3's home.

Couple 3 separates, couple 1 walks through, dividing them.
The first girl returns to her home position, her partner walks left. They meet and elbow swing.

All boys swing their corner ladies.

Promenade with the corner back to boy's home.

The first boy repeats all above with a new partner.
Second boy does it twice. Third and fourth boy do it twice.

(Use any ending call. End with allemande left and grand right and left again.)

Texas Star

Music: Any square dance arrangement of "Cripple Creek."

Ladies to the center, and back to the bar.

Gents to the center and form a star,
With your right hand across,
Now, back with your left, and don't get lost.

Man takes his partner's right hand and twirls her into the center, then out again.
Men catch right hands and move clockwise.
Men pivot, catch left hands, and move counterclockwise.

Meet your partner and pass her by,
Pick up the next girl on the fly.

Each man passes his partner and hooks elbows with his right hand lady. He is still holding his opposite's left hand in the center.

Ladies swing in, and the gents swing out.
Turn that Texas Star about.

Men drop left hands and swing the ladies to the inside. Ladies star with right hands across. The set is still moving.

Now, do-si-do, and a little more do,
Swing your partner and promenade home.

The man releases the elbow hook. He takes his lady's left hand in his left hand and swings her until she faces the corner. The do-si-do continues as usual.

Wagon Wheel

Music: Any square dance arrangement.

First couple, balance, first couple swing. Out to the couple at the right of the ring and circle four.

Self-explanatory.

Leave that girl, go on to the next and circle three.

Lady No. 1 stays with couple 2; man No. 1 goes on to couple 3 and circles three. No. 2 man hooks elbows with his partner and lady 1; they stand facing center.

Steal that girl like honey from a bee, put her on your right.

Lead man takes lady No. 3 as he advances to couple 4.

And on to the next and circle four.

Man No. 1 and lady No. 3 circle with couple 4.

Leave that girl, and go home alone.

Man No. 1 returns to his home position alone. No. 4 gent hooks elbows with his partner and lady 3.

Forward six, and back to the bar.

Men 2 and 4 and their ladies take 4 steps to the center then return to place.

End men forward and back like a shooting star.

Men 1 and 3 move forward, then back.

Forward six, and sashay 'round as you cross over.

Men 2 and 4 again move to center, catch hands, and turn half way round; so that when they go back to place they will be on the opposite side of the square.

End men go on to Dover.

Men 1 and 3 meet at the center, twirl half around and back into place.

Now right hand up and left hand under.

Men 2 and 4 take the ladies' hands then raise right arms and twirl the right hand lady (partner) to the man on the left, and the left hand lady to the man on the right. The right hand lady moves first.

Now men 2 and 4 become the "end men." The dance is continued three times until everyone has his original partner.

Sioux City Sue

Music: The tune "Sioux City Sue" or the recorded singing call.

Swing, boys, swing. Everybody swing.   Swing twice around.
Promenade around the ring.
Promenade back home again,
Just like you always do.
Everybody swing, now swing Sioux City   Again swing twice.
Sue.
First couple right and circle four hands   1st couple leads to 2nd couple and
'round.   circles once around.
Dos-a-dos your opposite, the lady once   Sashay the opposite lady, returning to
around.   original position.
Dos-a-dos your partner, and you swing   Sashay your partner.
her too.
Both couples swing. Now swing Sioux   Swing your partner twice around with
City Sue.   a waist swing.
On to the next, and you circle four   The figure is repeated until couple 1
hands 'round.   returns home. Then the introduction
is repeated, and couples 2, 3, and 4
each lead a complete figure.

Rose of San Antone [1]

Music: The Tune of "San Antonio Rose" or the recorded singing call.

Opener.
Oh, you swing 'em, boys,   Self-explanatory.
You swing 'em 'round and 'round.
Promenade that little lady
All around the town.
Promenade back home
With the one you call your own,
And swing with the Rose of San An-
tone.
Figure.
First couple right, and you circle four   Couples 1 and 2 circle once around.
and smile.
Now dos-a-dos your partner in that   Each man takes his partner's left hand
good ole mountain style.   in his right hand, leads her around
in front of him and around him until
she is back on his right. The man
does not change the direction he is
facing and does not release his partner's hand. (The man may well pre-
tend he is twirling a lasso.)
Swing with your opposites until you   Each man swings his opposite lady once
find your own.   around.
Then swing with the Rose of San An-   Each man swings his partner.
tone.

Couple 1 leads on to the next until they have danced with all the couples. Between figures the following chorus is danced:

---

[1] Composer: Dr. J. Vannes Boone, Dallas, Texas.

Chorus:

All gents swing your corners, the lady
   on your left.
Go back and swing your own; she's the
   one you love the best.
Allemande left your corners,
And dos-a-dos your own.
Balance to your partner, and weave
   that ring back home.
Now you weave that ring,
Go 'round and 'round.
And when you meet your partner,
You will dos-a-dos around.
You weave that ring, until you find
   your own.
Then swing with that Rose of San
   Antone.

To "weave the ring" the dancers pass
their partners' right shoulders, then
continue around the set doing a
grand right and left without touching hands. The men fold their arms
across their chests, and the ladies
catch their skirts in their hands.

Sashay your partner and continue moving in the same direction as before.
When you meet your partner, you will
be at home position. Swing her once
around.

Repeat the entire dance until all four couples have been the lead couple.

Alabama Jubilee

     Music: "Alabama Jubilee." [2]

Four little ladies promenade
The inside of the ring.
Back to your partner,
And give him a swing.
Dos-a-dos your corner,
Just once around.
Bow to your partner now,
Swing him 'round and 'round.
Four men promenade
The inside of the hall.
Back to your partner,
And dos-a-dos all.
The corner girl will swing with you.
And promenade like an old shoo-shoo.
To the Alabama Jubilee.

Ladies go into the center and move to
the right until they return home.

Ladies sashay their corner men.

Men move in a circle to the right.

Men sashay their partners.

Each man swings his corner lady.
Each man promenades his corner until
the next call comes for four little
ladies to promenade. Couples should
not try to get home before the next
figure begins.

Repeat the figure three times until each person has his original partner.

Mixer (as called by Joe Lewis)
All join hands and circle left,
And form that big old ring.
Break the ring with a corner swing,
Leave her on your right, and you're
   gone again.
Ring, ring, a pretty little ring,
Break it again with a corner swing,

---

[2] Singing call recorded by Joe Lewis, Dallas, Texas, the composer of this dance.

Leave her on your right, and circle—
And don't you know.

Do-si-do, and a little more do,
Like a chicken in the bread pan
   a'peckin' out dough.
When you get back home this time,
It's stop, you know.
Go all around your left-hand lady,
See-saw 'round that taw.
Allemande left with that old left hand,
Partner right and a right and left
   grand.
Here comes Sal, here comes Sue,
And here comes the gal that came with
   you.
Take them home on the old shoo-shoo.
Promenade around that ring,
Get 'em happy, give 'em a swing.
To the Alabama Jubilee.

Swannee River
(Only the opener of this dance is sung to the tune "Swannee River." The dance is recorded as a singing call, but it may be used as a patter call, with singing only during the opener.)

Opener.
Allemande left, and a grand right and left. SING:
"Way down upon the Swannee River
Far, far, away.
There's where my heart am longing ever,
Down where the old folks stay."

When partners meet half around the set, they hold right hands and step left and "kick," then step, kick right in time with the rhythm of the song. Then they pass right shoulders again with their partner and continue the grand right and left until they are back at home position.

Figure.
(First couple)
Lady go 'round the lady
And the gent go 'round the gent.

1st couple moves to face couple 2. Lady 1 goes between couple 2 and circles lady 2 without changing the direction she faces.
Man 1 follows his lady and circles man 2 back to place.

The gent go 'round the lady
And the lady 'round the gent.
Circle half, and right and left through.

The man moves in a circle around lady 2, then the lady goes around the man.
Circle four until couple 1 is facing the center of the set. (The couples simply change positions.) Each lady gives her right hand to the opposite man. They pass right shoulders and meet their partners again.

Swing your partner once around
And take her on with you.

Couples 1 and 2 swing. Couple 1 swings toward the center of the set to be ready to go on to the next.

And the lady go 'round the lady, etc.

Repeat figure until No. 1 couple has danced with couples 3 and 4. The entire dance including the opener is danced three more times for couples 2, 3, and 4 to lead.

Folk Dance

Kalvelis

Record: Sonart Folk Dance Album I-Folkraft 1051A (Lithuanian-Blacksmith).

Formation: About eight couples form single circle facing counterclockwise.

Step 1. All polka (without hop) eight steps right.	Measure:	1–8
All polka (without hop) eight steps left.	Measure:	1–8
Chorus. Clap own hands; partner's right; own hands; partner's left. Double hand grasp and skip to left four times; skip to right four times.	Measure:	9–16
Repeat.	Measure:	9–16
Step 2. Girls do four polka steps into circle, turn, and four	Measure:	1–8
polka steps back to place. Boys do same.	Measure:	1–8
Chorus (twice)	Measure:	9–16
Step 3. Girls weave around circle going back of the first	Measure:	1–16
dancer and in front of the next, etc.; sixteen polka steps.		
Boys do same.	Measure:	1–16
Chorus.		
Step 4. All do grand right and left.	Measure:	1–16
Chorus (twice)	Measure:	1–16
Step 5. All join hands and polka eight times right as in	Measure:	1–8
Step 1.		
Polka eight times left.	Measure:	1–8

Tantoli

Simple Version: Crampton, *The Folk Dance Book*—Record (Scandinavian).

Formation: Couples in double circle facing counterclockwise with inside hands joined and free hands on hips.

Step 1. With outside foot, each couple places heel to floor forward, and toe on floor backward. Polka step hopping on inside foot.	Measure:	1
Repeat three times, beginning on inside foot, outside, and inside.	Measure:	2
	Measure:	3–8
Step 2. Partners face, join hands at shoulder level and turn clockwise with sixteen step hops, boy starting on left foot; girl on right.	Measure:	8

(This step has been called the "Windmill" because the arms are lowered toward the foot that the hop is taken on and raised on the opposite side.)

Repeat dance.

Csebogar

Record: Victor 20992; Folkraft 1196 (Hungarian).

Formation: Partners form single circle facing in; girl on boy's right; hands joined.

Step 1. All move clockwise with eight slides.	Measure: 1–4
Step 2. All move counterclockwise with eight slides.	Measure: 5–8
Step 3. Hands still joined and held high; take four skips toward center of circle.	Measure: 9–10
Lower hands; skip backward to original places.	Measure: 11–12
Step 4. Partners face and place right arm around partner's waist and raise left arm high, with elbow straight. Skip eight times turning clockwise.	Measure: 13–16

(*Variation*—Upper grades may use eight paddle steps, or the Hungarian. Turn twice, around with a hop right, step left, and step right.)

Step 5. All face partners; join both hands and step sideways toward center of circle, closing with opposite foot in four slow slides, or draws.	Measure: 17–20
Repeat to outside of circle.	Measure: 21–24
Step 6. Repeat action of Step 5 with two draw steps.	Measure: 25–28
Step 7. Repeat Step 4.	Measure: 29–32

Gustaf's Skoal

Record: Victor 20988; Folkraft 1175 (Swedish). ("Skoal" means formal greeting.)

Formation: Square, four couples.

1. Head couples—three steps forward and bow on 4th count.	Measure: 1–2
2. Head couples—three steps backward and feet together on 4th count.	Measure: 3–4
3. Side couples do same.	Measure: 5–8
4. Repeat all.	Measure: 1–8
5. Side couples join inside hands and form arch. Head couples skip toward each other, take new partners. Skip through arch, girls go to right, boys to left. Leave new partners and return to original positions meeting own partners.	Measure: 9–12
6. All clap hands, join both hands with partner and make one complete turn.	Measure: 13–16
7. Side couples repeat Step 5 with head couples forming arch. All repeat Step 6.	Measure: 9–16

Danish Dance of Greeting

Record: Victor 17158; Folkraft 1187.

Formation: Single circle; dancers facing the center with hands on hips.

Step 1. Clap hands twice; turn to partner and bow. Clap hands twice; turn and bow to neighbor.	Measure: 1–2
Step 2. Stamp right; stamp left; turn in place four running steps.	Measure: 3–4
Repeat measures 1 and 2.	Measure: 1–4
Step 3. All join hands and take sixteen running steps to right.	Measure: 5–8
Repeat to left. Repeat entire dance.	Measure: 9–16

Chimes of Dunkirk

Record: World of Fun Series, M 105 (French, Flemish, Belgian).

Formation: Double circle of partners facing each other; boys with back to center of circle.

Step 1. Clap three times; pause.	Measure: 1–4
Step 2. Partners join both hands and walk around circle in eight counts.	Measure: 5–8
Step 3. Partners join right hands and balance. Repeat.	Measure: 9–12
Step 4. Partners walk around each other once and boy moves on to his left to the next girl.	Measure: 13–16

Ace of Diamonds

Record: Victor 20989; World of Fun Series, M 102 (Danish).

Formation: Double circle; partners facing; boys with back to center of circle.

Step 1. Partners clap hands once; stamp foot once; hook right arms and swing around once.	Measure: 1–4
Repeat using left arm.	Measure: 5–8
Step 2. Girl puts hands on hips and moves backward toward center of circle with a step, hop. Step left; hop left; step right; hop right. Repeat. Boy follows with arms crossed on chest: step right; hop right; step right; hop right. Repeat. Return in reverse.	Measure: 9–16
Step 3. Polka—skating position, going counterclockwise.	Measure: 1–16

Troika

Record: Kismet S112; Folkraft 1170 (Russian).

Formation: Groups of three facing counterclockwise. Center dancer is a boy, outside dancers girls. Hands are joined; free hand on hips.

Figure I

Step 1. Four running steps forward diagonally to right.	Measure: 1
Step 2. Repeat diagonally to left.	Measure: 2
Step 3. Eight running steps forward around circle.	Measure: 3–4
Step 4. Hands still joined, the girl on the boy's right runs under arch, made by boy and girl on left, in eight steps. Other two run in place.	Measure: 5–6
Step 5. Girl on left runs under arch and back to place in eight steps.	Measure: 7–8

Figure II

Step 1. Each group of three joins hands in a circle and runs to left (clockwise) for twelve steps, beginning on left foot.	Measure: 9–11
Step 2. Stamp in place—left; right; left	Measure: 12
Repeat steps 1 and 2 running to right (counterclockwise).	Measure: 13–16
Release hands and repeat entire dance with same partners. Partners may change in measure 16. Girls raise outside hands to make an arch, release boy and he runs with four steps to next group while girls stamp in place.	Measure: 16

Green Sleeves

Record: [3] Folk Fun Funfest (Dick Kraus) (English).

Formation: Double circle in sets of two couples, numbered 1 and 2, facing counterclockwise; girls on right.

Step 1. Holding hands, walk forward sixteen steps.

Step 2. Form a star in sets. Man No. 1 gives hand to girl No. 2 and man No. 2 to girl No. 1. Walk clockwise eight steps; change to left hands and walk back to place counterclockwise.

Step 3. Couple No. 1 join hands and back under arch made by couple No. 2 who walk forward four steps, then walk backward while No. 1 makes the arch. Repeat. Repeat entire dance.

Tropanka

Folk Dancer Record: Disc Album 635 (Bulgarian stamping dance).

Formation: Single circle; little fingers joined.

Stamping step: Cross foot over in front in ballet position with heel turned out.

Step 1. Beginning on right foot, take five running steps to right and stamp twice with left foot. Turn and run to left five steps and stamp twice with right foot.	Measure: 1–2
	Measure: 3–4
Repeat first four measures.	Measure: 1–4
Step 2. Facing center, all step on right foot, hop on right foot and swing left foot in front. Step; hop; swing; starting on left foot.	Measure: 5
Step on right foot; cross left foot over and stamp twice.	Measure: 6
Repeat measures 5 and 6, starting on left foot.	Measure: 7–8
Repeat measures.	Measure: 5–8
Step 3. Moving toward center of circle, all starting on right foot, step, hop right, step, and hop left. Step right and stamp twice with left foot. (Arms raised high, shout "Hey!")	Measure: 5
	Measure: 6

Repeat action of measures 5 and 6, dancing backward, starting with left foot. Gradually lower arms.

Repeat measures 9 through 16 as in measures 1 through 8.

The Crested Hen

Record: Folkraft 1194 (Danish).[4]

Formation: Sets of three, one boy with a girl on either side.

Step: The hop-step is done through the entire dance. Step on left foot on count one; hop on left foot; swing right foot in front of it on count two, keeping the knee bent. Reverse and step-hop on right foot; swing left foot to front.

Figure 1. All sets of 3's join hands to form circles. Moving to left (clockwise) stamp left foot and do eight step-hops.	Measure: 1–8

---

3 Educational Dance Recordings, P.O. Box 6062, Bridgeport, Ct. 06606.

4 N. P. Neilson and Winifred Van Hagen: *Physical Education for Elementary Schools.* New York, A. S. Barnes & Co., 1929.

Dancers lean back as they circle.

Repeat measures 1 to 8, moving counterclockwise with   Measure: 1–8
eight step-hops.

Figure 2. Girls release hands and place free hands on hips.   Measure: 9–12
Boy never releases the hands. Girl at the left of boy dances
(step-hops) in front of him and under the arch made by
raised hands of the boy and the girl on the right.

Repeat same action with girl on the right, passing through   Measure: 13–16
arch.

Mayim [5] (Water)

Record: Folkraft 1108a (Israeli).

Formation: Students stand in circle facing center, hands joined and down.

1. Four circasia combinations to the left. For each circasia combination:
   a. Place right foot in front and across left (accent right foot).
   b. Bring left foot alongside right foot.
   c. Place right foot back, across left foot, to left.
   d. Hop on left foot alongside right foot.
2. All take 8 steps toward center of circle, lifting hands gradually, accentuating first step by raising right knee.
3. All face left and take four walking steps toward left, starting with right foot.
4. While hopping on right foot, tap with left foot over right foot. Then tap with left foot to the left side. This combination is done 4 times.
5. While hopping on left foot, tap right foot over left foot. Then tap with right foot to right side. Slap hands on odd beat. This combination is done 4 times.

This dance is supposed to convey the movement of water, of waves, of going toward the well, and the joy of discovering water in an arid country.

Raatikko

Folk Dancer Record: Scandinavian: 1123 (Finnish Polka—Old Maid's Dance).

Formation: Couple; social dance position.

Step 1. Eight polka steps, turning clockwise.

Step 2. Four draw steps. Boy has girl by one arm pulling and girl moves reluctantly toward rock.

Step 3. Eight slide steps away from rock.

Step 4. Repeat steps 2 and 3.

Repeat all.

Background: On the coast of Finland, there is a large rock close to the beach. According to the story, if a boy succeeds in pulling a girl behind the rock, she will be an old maid.

Gie Gordon's

Beltona Record: BL-2455; Folkraft 1162 (Scotch—The Gay Gordons).

Formation: Couples in varsouvienne position (couples facing same direc-

---

[5] Maine Folk Dance Camp. Contributed by the Michael Hermans.

tion; boy's right arm across back to girl's right shoulder and holding her right hand at shoulder level; left hands joined in front).

Step 1. Both start on left foot. Take four walking steps forward. Reverse and take four walking steps backward, but continue in the same line of direction. Repeat.

Step 2. Boy holds girl's right hand high with his right hand and polkas forward as girl does four polkas (clockwise) turning under boy's arm.

Step 3. In social dance position, do four polka steps turning clockwise. Repeat entire dance.

Finger Polka

Standard Record: 2001A (Lithuanian).

Formation: Couples form double circle, facing counterclockwise; boys on inside of circle.

Step 1. Eight polka steps in open position (hold inside hands, starting hop on outside foot, etc., back to back and face to face).

Step 2. Eight polka steps in closed position turning clockwise.

Step 3. Drop hands and face partner. Stamp three times; clap own hands three times. Repeat. Shake right finger at partner; make turn on own left, slapping right hand against partner's right hand as turn is taken. Stamp three times. Repeat entire dance.

Road To The Isles

Record: Imperial 1005A (Scotch).

Formation: Couples in varsouvienne position.

Step 1. Point left toe forward and hold. Grapevine step moving to right. Step left foot back of right foot; step right to side; step left foot in front of right foot and hold.	Measure: 1 Measure: 2–3
Point right toe forward and hold, and grapevine to left stepping right, left, right and hold.	Measure: 4 Measure: 5–6
Point left toe forward and hold.	Measure: 7
Point left toe backward in deep dip and hold.	Measure: 8
Step 2. Schottische forward diagonally to left, beginning on left foot—left; right; left; hop.	Measure: 9–10
Schottische forward diagonally to right, beginning on right foot—right; left; right; hop. On hop, in measure 12, half turn to right facing in opposite direction, keeping hands joined.	Measure: 11–12
Schottische, beginning on left foot. On hop, take half turn to left facing original direction. In place, step right; left; right; hold.	Measure: 13–14 Measure: 15–16

Bleking

Record: Victor 20989; Folkraft 1188 (Swedish).

Formation: Partners face with both hands joined.

Step 1. Bleking (Blē-king): Jump lightly to left foot, placing right heel to floor—count 1. See-saw arms by extending right arm forward with elbow straight and left arm backward with elbow bent. Reverse arms and jump lightly on right foot, placing left heel to floor—count 2.	Measure: 1

Repeat Bleking step three times in quick time—count   Measure: 2
1 and 2.
Repeat measures 1–2 three times.   Measure: 3–8
Step 2. Extend arms sideward and turn in clockwise   Measure: 9–16
direction with sixteen step-hops, alternately raising and
lowering arms and kicking free leg to the side of the hops.
Repeat entire dance.

SUGGESTED READINGS

ANDREWS, GLADYS, *Creative Rhythmic Movement for Children.* Englewood Cliffs,
    N.J.: Prentice-Hall, 1974.

HALL, TILMAN, *Dance.* Belmont, Cal.: Wadsworth, 1974.

MYNATT, CONSTANCE, and BERNARD KAIMAN, *Folk Dancing for Students and
    Teachers.* Dubuque, Iowa: Brown, 1968.

SHURR, EVELYN, *Movement Experiences for Children.* New York: Appleton-
    Century-Crofts, 1967.

SMITH, RAYMOND, *Square Dance Handbook and Collection of Square Dances and
    Mixers.* 1038 Cedar Hill, Dallas, Texas.

SPIESMAN, MILDRED, *Folk Dancing.* Philadelphia: W. B. Saunders, 1970.

VANNIER, MARYHELEN, and HOLLIS FAIT, *Teaching Physical Education in Sec-
    ondary Schools,* 4th ed. Philadelphia: W. B. Saunders, 1975.

Suggested Records For Movement Exploration

BURNS, JOSEPH, and EDITH WHEELER, *Creative Rhythm Album* (Visit to a farm,
    park, and circus), Stanley Bowmar Company, Inc., 12 Cleveland Street,
    Valhalla, N.Y. 10595.

CARR, DOROTHY, and BRYANT CRATTY, *Listening and Moving,* Educational Activ-
    ities, Freeport, N.Y.

Chicken Fat—Capitol CF1000.

JERVEY, ARDEN, and DOROTHY CARR, *Simplified Folk Dance Favorites for Excep-
    tional Children,* Educational Activities, Freeport, N.Y. 11520.

McCORMACK, MARIE, *Songs and Games of Physical Education for Boys and Girls,*
    Golden LP Record LP114.

Music for Creative Pre-Schoolers, Q.T. Records, 73 Fifth Ave., N.Y. 10003.

Play and Learn, Summit Industries, P.O. Box 415, Highland Park, Ill. 60035.

15

Camping and Outdoor Education

Camps for handicapped people have become increasingly common in the last decade. Scattered throughout the nation are camps for those with particular disabilities such as cardiac disorders, orthopedic handicaps, diabetes, and epilepsy. There are also camps for the blind, the mentally retarded, and the deaf. Outstanding camping programs are conducted at the Timber Trail Camp for Crippled Children in Aconomowoc, Wisconsin, the Bay Cliff Health Camp in Big Bay, Michigan, and the Lions Club Camp for Crippled Children in Kerville, Texas. In the east, Camp Wapanacki, sponsored by the New York Institute for Blind Children of New York City, and Camp Emanuel, sponsored by the Jewish Institute for the Education of Handicapped are conducting excellent camps for the atypical.[1]

Although camping provides opportunities to become acquainted with the wonders of nature and new experiences, its values to the handicapped are notable. Through camping, people can learn many new and important physical and social skills—from learning to fish to discovering how to get along with peers.

---

[1] See the 1976 edition of *The Directory of Approved Camps,* American Camping Association, Bradford Woods, Martinsville, Ind. 46151, for a complete list of nationally recognized camps for the handicapped. Also see the *Directory of Camps for the Handicapped,* National Easter Seal Society, 2023 W. Odgen Avenue, Chicago, Illinois, 60612.

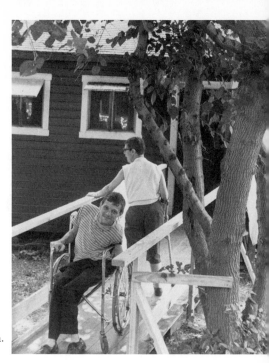

The camp should be in a wooded area.
Courtesy of the AAHPER.

THE CAMP SITE AND GROUNDS

Ideally, a camp for the handicapped should be located in a wooded area close to nature, yet near enough to a town or city so that transportation is no problem. It should have sufficient outdoor space (a minimum of 200 square feet per child) so that children can run and play out-of-doors safely. There should be an unused borderland for a "buffer zone" that is either fenced off or has natural barriers.

Swimming and boating areas should be fenced off. A swimming pool with graduated depths is preferable to a sandy beach. There should also be sprinklers and wading pools on the camp property. Other musts include:

1. A large number of shade trees
2. One toilet for every 10 persons
3. A safe water supply
4. Available medical services nearby
5. Indoor space for rainy days (at least 35 square feet per camper)
6. Shelters or pavilions
7. Sleeping quarters
8. Eating and cooking areas
9. Refrigeration for perishable foods

The camp site, facilities, leadership, and program should all meet the standards of the American Camping Association[2] and be periodically

---

[2] Available from the American Camping Association, Bradford Woods, Martinsville, Ind. 46151.

inspected by a visiting evaluative team from this association as well as by visiting teams from the state board of health.

THE CAMP PROGRAM

Camp programs should be geared to fit all age groups. Young adults, middle-aged groups, and even the aged are becoming increasingly enthusiastic about camping. Although program activities for older disabled people are apt to be less strenuous than those for children, they should revolve for the most part around food, shelter, and recreation in the out-of-doors.

The best camp programs are counselor-camper made. Care should be taken not to duplicate activities the campers could do just as easily at home or on a playground. Recreational sports such as baseball and tennis belong more to the city, whereas canoeing and outdoor cooking are best suited for camp. Because camping offers a unique kind of recreational opportunity, care should be taken to build the program around activities that can be done better at camp than elsewhere. This holds true for camps for the handicapped as well as for the normal.

Counselor-camper planned programs offer opportunities for adults and youth to learn to contribute, share, and respect one another. It is necessary, however, that the director and staff plan program possibilities before they present them to the campers. Here children gain valuable experiences in learning the techniques of group planning; because they share in selecting and conducting what they wish to do, activities are done *with* them, not *for* them.

So that the greatest benefits may accrue from counselor-camper planning, program possibilities should be explored to determine what activities can best be done in the particular camp environment with a particular type of camper in mind (blind, deaf, retarded, etc.). Such exploration might include the following questions:

1. Are the selected activities fun to do?
2. Can both campers and counselors assume responsibility for carrying out the selected activities?
3. Are the selected activities based upon the needs, interests, and capacities of the group?
4. What opportunities are provided in carrying out the activities for growth in skills and appreciations?
5. How will the selected activities lead to a better use of present and future leisure time?
6. What are the opportunities for the development of individual and group creative expression?
7. Will the selected activities develop moral and ethical values?
8. Will the selected activities contribute to the development of each individual who takes part?
9. Will the selected activities make best use of time, facilities, groups, community resources, and staff?

10. Are the activities scheduled or arranged so that there is a tapering off, with less strenuous ones near the end of the day?
11. Is the program elastic, flexible, and modifiable?

Suggested camping program areas include:

Astronomy	Gardening
Explorations	Lashing
Excursions	Nature hikes, trails, study
Cookouts	Map and compass reading and
Carpentry	construction
Fire building	Outdoor cooking and menu planning
Fishing	Overnight hikes
Hiking	Outdoor shelter construction
Hunting	Use of camp tools

If the camp is conducted on the basis of overnight, weekend, weekly, or longer duration, the evening recreational program should be made up of activities not done during the day. These might include such activities as:

Amateur night	Parties
Banquets	birthday
Masquerades	costume
Pageants	seasonal
Community business	Game nights
camp post office	Indian pow-wows or council rings
camp bank	Moonlight hikes
camp store	Scavenger hunts
Discussion groups	Square and folk dancing
Firelighting ceremonials	Tournaments
Hobby clubs	Treasure hunts
World friendship nights	Corn roasts or clambakes

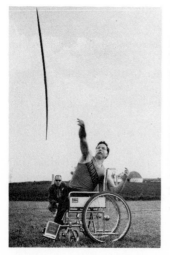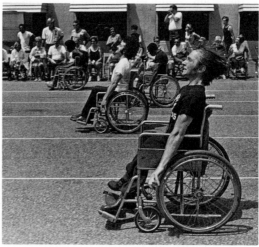

A track meet can be an ideal camp activity, too. Courtesy of the AAHPER.

Children come to camp primarily because of the program. They want it to be adventurous, fun, thrilling, and made up of new as well as traditional activities. Everything done at camp, from clean-up duties to crafts, is equally important from an educational standpoint.

Directors customarily break down the complete program into the following classifications and sub-groups:

1. The Daily Program
   a. Athletic activities
      Team sports
      Individual sports
      Aquatic sports
      Land sports
   b. Health-related activities
      Camp feeding
      Clean-up duties
      Rest hours
   c. Creative arts
      Arts and crafts
      Dance
      Dramatics
      Music
   d. Campcraft activities
      Hiking
      Outdoor cooking
      Outdoor living
      Map construction and reading
      Land conservation
      Nature lore
2. Evening Recreation Program
      Competitive games
      Parties, plays, and pantomimes
      Club, interest, and hobby groups
      Leisure-time activities
3. Special Events
   a. Canoe trips
      Cookout trips
      Hikes
      Boat trips
      Mountain-climbing trips
      Pack-mule or horseback trips
      Sailing trips
      Visits to local industries
      Visits to places of interest in the community
   b. Guest speakers or outside entertainers
      Visiting days
4. Moral or Religious Program
   a. Daily worship or ceremonials
      Grace before meals
      Group discussions
      Flag ceremonials
   b. Weekly worship program

Camp programs vary widely throughout the country. Factors causing this variation are (1) philosophy, aims, goals, and objectives of the
camp; (2) surroundings and climatic conditions; (3) organization of the
camp (centralized or decentralized); (4) camper age range; (5) camper
experience and home background; and (6) leadership skills.

Some camps are glorified playgrounds and summer resorts, where
the program is made up largely of activities duplicating those found in
cities. In these, highly organized sports, arts and craft programs patterned
after school activities, and other transplanted recreational games have
crowded out activities best suited for the natural camp environment. On
the other hand, many camps believe in providing as many of the unique
out-of-doors programs as possible; these are geared to teach people the
fundamental skills of nature, campcraft and outdoor living. In these, all
phases of living connected with the out-of-doors, with a nature-oriented
creative arts program utilizing natural resources, form basic program
materials.

Camp programs are built by two methods—by adults entirely, or
by counselor-camper planning committees.

Types of Programs

There are three types of programs found in camps: (1) those that
are highly scheduled or compartmentalized, (2) those that involve se-
lective choice, and (3) those that are built around learning to live in
and enjoy the out-of-doors.

The highly scheduled type of program chops up the camper's day
into hourly activities. Bells or bugles signal the end of one activity and
the beginning of another. Campers scurry from one class to another in
much the same fashion as a formal school. Little choice is given to elect
activities most appealing to campers. Each child falls into a tightly
scheduled pattern geared to his age or unit group. A typical program
patterned after this plan might look like this:

7:00	Reveille
8:00	Breakfast
8:30–9:00	Clean-up duties
9:00–10:00	First-period classes
10:00–11:00	Second-period classes
11:00–12:00	Swimming for everyone
12:00–12:30	Free time, meetings, or tournament play
12:30–1:30	Dinner
1:30–2:30	Rest hour
2:30–3:30	Third-period classes
3:30–4:30	Fourth-period classes
4:30–5:30	Fifth-period classes
5:30–6:00	Supervised free play
6:00–7:00	Supper
7:00–7:30	Camp store, meetings, or tournament play
7:30–8:30	Evening recreational program
9:00	Taps

Selective-choice programs are found in more progressive camps. Here campers select activities in which they wish to participate weekly, daily, or for the entire season. Definite times are set for retiring, meals, and rest hours. Swimming is usually required of all. Freedom is customarily given to select one individual or team sport, one creative activity, and one campcraft activity. The daily schedule might look like this:

7:30	Reveille
8:00	Breakfast
8:30–9:00	Clean-up duties
9:00–10:00	Individual or team sports
10:00–11:00	Creative activities
11:00–12:00	Swimming
12:00–1.00	Free time
1:00–2:00	Dinner
2:00–3:00	Rest hour
3:00–4:00	Campcraft activities
4:00–5:00	Creative activities or individual sports
5:00–6:00	Supervised free play
6:00–7:00	Supper
7:00–7:30	Canteen, meetings, or free time
7:30–8:30	Evening recreational program
9:00	Taps

Programs built around learning to live in the out-of-doors generally only contain set times for rising and retiring, rest hour, and meal time. Within these limits, activities are devised by campers and counselors around the problems that arise from outdoor living. The entire program is bent upon providing purposeful experiences in which learning is achieved through life situations. Such a program would be something like this:

7:00	Reveille
7:30–8:30	Preparation and eating breakfast
8:30–9:30	Camp clean-up duties
9:30–11:30	Exploration activities, planning the day's events
11:30–1:00	Preparation and eating dinner
1:00–2:00	Rest hour
2:00–5:00	Exploration activities, camp projects, utilizing campcraft skills
5:00–5:30	Leisure time
5:30–7:00	Preparation and eating supper
7:00–7:30	Camp business (handled entirely by campers)
7:30–9:00	Evening program
9:00	Taps

Suggestions for Improving Camp Programs

If camping is to realize the educational potentialities it holds for youth, serious consideration must be given to the type of program the camp is to offer, how it is to be planned and conducted, and how it is to be evaluated.

If one accepts the thesis that camping is a unique type of group living and education that takes place while living close to nature in the out-of-doors, it becomes apparent that directors, counselors, and campers must seriously consider those things that are the unique offerings of the camp environment and that are the most useful in education. The thesis is that those things that can best be learned in the classroom should be learned there, but those things that can best be learned only out in the open should be fully utilized while in the camp environment. Directors who follow this thinking often include in their programs such activities as starting and running weather stations, marking trails, exploring, outdoor cooking, excursions to nearby points of interest, making things from natural resources, spiritual appreciation experiences, and concerns involved with ecology.

Day Camps

Most recreation departments offer summer programs for children in day camps. Many hold these programs on their own playgrounds; others take the children to nearby lakes, mountains, or wooded areas for a day of outdoor fun and challenges. The best of such camps provide children with exciting and adventurous activities they can only do in a camp setting. They also introduce the child to the many mysteries of the world of nature. The most successful day camp directors believe in planning with children a program that omits the many activities that can be done elsewhere and includes only those they can best do through a camping program.

Such programs are greatly needed in large metropolitan areas where many children are missing the thrill of being close to nature and growing things. However, many living in rural small towns can profit greatly from being, working, and playing with other children through such a camp program. Obviously, such a camp can benefit the atypical, as well as the normal child.

BASIC CAMPCRAFT SKILLS

Basic camp skills should be taught to all youth and adults who go to camp, including the handicapped. Some of these can be taught before the camping adventure, in community centers, at Scout meetings, or in special classes. Such pre-training can be especially meaningful and valuable for disabled individuals.

Teaching of Basic Skills

FIRE BUILDING

A fire in camp is used for cooking, warmth, protection from animals, and companionship. Storytelling, visiting with friends, special programs, and just plain daydreaming are experiences that come to mean more

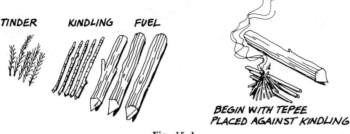

TINDER   KINDLING   FUEL

BEGIN WITH TEPEE
PLACED AGAINST KINDLING

Fig. 15–1

when a person is close to a campfire in a joyful outdoor living experience.

Select a campfire site away from trees and bushes. Build the fire with the wind at your back. Start with tinder of small dry twigs (Figure 15–1). Have other wood gathered and ready for use. Add larger twigs gradually as the fire burns. Use soft wood (pines, spruces, cedars, aspen, etc.) for quick, hot boiling fires. Hard wood (oak, hickory, maple, etc.) makes the best slow-burning fire. When building a fire remember to

1. Build it so that air can reach the tinder and fuel (air coming from the bottom or side is best)
2. Arrange the wood so that the flames will travel from piece to piece
3. Use for tinder small, dry sticks, dried grass, or tree bark that snaps into small pieces readily
4. Gradually increase the size of the wood, after getting the tinder started, to build the fire higher
5. Use split wood for kindling, if possible (it burns faster)
6. Have all fuel ready before you light the fire
7. Be sure your campfire is out before leaving it

Remember, even handicapped people must learn safety procedures for camping activities they are able to participate in. Also it is best for them to do as much for and by themselves as they can. In many cases, as has been mentioned, it is well to pair those who are more disabled with people who are less handicapped—for the benefits of *helping* are often equal to those of being helped.

OUTDOOR COOKING

Fire-building progression should be linked with cooking (Figure 15–2). Outdoor cooking can be a challenge to both the novice and the skilled chef. For the handicapped, especially, it is a useful skill that can also add to a general feeling of accomplishment and competence.

One-Pot Meals	Steak
Chili	Desserts
Baked beans	Biscuits
Stew	Fish
Chowder	Chops
Baking	Bean hole
Plank	Cooked cereals

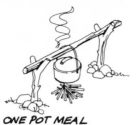  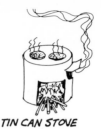

ONE POT MEAL   COOK OVER COALS   TIN CAN STOVE

Fig. 15–2 Outdoor Cooking Methods and Fires

Beans	Baked meats
Potatoes	Reflector oven
Baked meats	Cookies
Coals	Cake
Potatoes	Biscuits
Corn roast	Baked meats
Pig in a blanket	

It is best to teach beginners to cook one or two simple things at first and to supplement the meal with sandwiches and fruit. Children enjoy progressing from toasting sandwiches to frying hamburgers on tin can stoves. Each camper, regardless of age or condition, will thrill to cooking his entire meal on a tin can stove, tennis racket broiler, or green stick. Adults will favor progressing from fried bacon and eggs to broiled steaks, roast corn, or barbecues. Both groups should first cook individually, next in small groups of three or four, and finally prepare some food (clambake, barbecue, etc.) for ten or more people. Some will want to practice their skills at public outdoor grills provided by local parks or at roadside fireplaces built beside state highways.

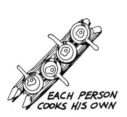 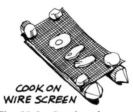 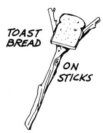

EACH PERSON COOKS HIS OWN   COOK ON WIRE SCREEN   TOAST BREAD ON STICKS

Fig. 15–2 *Continued*

Recipes

Campers will enjoy starting a collection of recipes for outdoor cooking as a hobby. Each leader who desires to teach others the fine art of outdoor cooking will find these recipes easy ones to learn:

Bread Twists. Add water according to directions to prepared biscuit dough or bisquick mix in a paper bag until a stiff dough is formed. Wind this around a green stick or a broom handle covered with foil, browning it slowly. Stuff holes with butter, bacon, or jam.

Pancakes. Add water to prepared mix. Have pan hot and well greased. Pour a spoonful on the pan. Cook until bubbles appear, turn. Add cinnamon, cooked rice, blueberries, or a cup of whole kernel canned corn to the batter for variety.

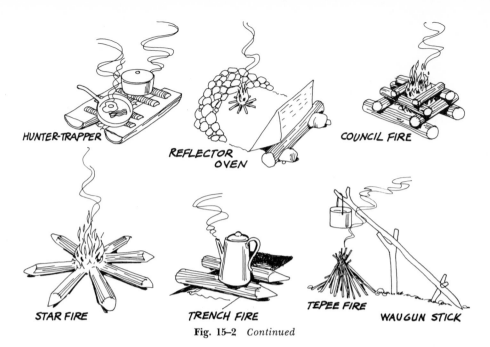

HUNTER-TRAPPER   REFLECTOR OVEN   COUNCIL FIRE

STAR FIRE   TRENCH FIRE   TEPEE FIRE   WAUGUN STICK

Fig. 15–2   *Continued*

Kabobs. Alternate cubes of beef (raw or partially cooked), potato, onion, carrot, and bacon on a green stick or pointed wire. Cook slowly over coals.

Roast Corn. Soak ears of corn in their husks in water for several hours. Cook in coals. Or wrap each water-soaked ear in aluminum foil after removing the husks. Cook in coals.

Chili Con Carne. Brown diced onions and hamburger. Combine and cook until done. Season with chili powder. Add one can of Mexican chili beans, one can of tomatoes, two tablespoons of catsup, and cook slowly.

S'mores. Make a sandwich of two white or graham crackers, add a piece of chocolate, a slice of apple, and one marshmallow. Toast slowly and sample. Judge for yourself whether you would like "S'more."

Baked Fish. Wrap a piece of frozen fillet in aluminum foil with a piece of raw carrot, potato, onion, and celery. Cook over coals.

Baked Chicken. As above, wrap your favorite piece of chicken in foil and cook with the vegetables.

Eggs in Mud. Cover eggs or potatoes with wet clay or mud. Cook 20 minutes in hot coals, potatoes one hour.

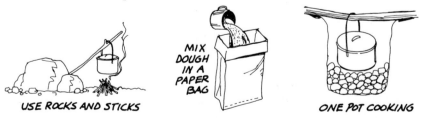

USE ROCKS AND STICKS   MIX DOUGH IN A PAPER BAG   ONE POT COOKING

Fig. 15–2   *Continued*

Potatoes Baked in Tin Can. Scrub potatoes and rub with butter or wrap in wax paper. Put in a large coffee can that has five holes punched in the top. Place in coals and pile them around the sides. Cook about one hour.

Pioneer Drumsticks. Mix chopped beef with onions, two eggs and one cup of crumbled corn flakes. Wrap this around the end of a green stick, squeezing it evenly in place. Cook over coals, turning frequently.

Camper's Stew. Have each person wrap the lower part of a large coffee can with foil. Put in alternate layers of chopped onions, carrots, celery, corn, and beef. Sprinkle tomato juice, canned tomatoes, or catsup over the top. Put on lid. Wrap the entire can with foil. Cook in hot coals for fifteen to twenty minutes.

Camp Coffee. Use one cup of cold water for every tablespoon of coffee. Put coffee in cloth bag, tying it loosely with string. Add to briskly boiling water and leave in for several minutes.

Camp Cocoa. Use one teaspoon of cocoa to every two of sugar. Add one cup of milk for every person, or four tablespoons of powdered milk to every cup of water, or a half cup of evaporated milk to every half cup of water. Mix cocoa and sugar with water in kettle and cook to a smooth paste. Add milk, a pinch of salt, and stir all together. Heat almost to a boil. Serve with a marshmallow for each cup.

AXE AND TOOL CRAFT

Hand Axe. Use for splitting firewood and cutting other small pieces of wood. Stand near a chopping block. Grasp the axe firmly. Slant the

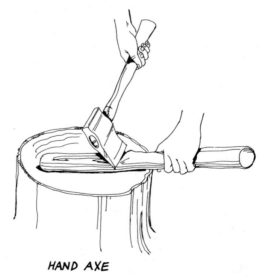

HAND AXE

Fig. 15–3

blade (Figure 15–3) to chop a large piece of wood so that it makes a V-shaped cut. To split wood, bite the axe blade into one end of the piece of wood or log. Raise the wood and axe together and bring them down sharply on a chopping block. Twist the axe against the wood to split it. To point a stick, hold it upright on the chopping block, strike it at an angle and turn it around. Cut down each new edge until you have a point.

Axe. Grasp the handle near the end with the left hand. Grip with the right hand about three-fourths of the way to the axe head. Raise the axe over the right shoulder (Figure 15–4a). As you bring it down sharply, slide the right hand down to meet the left one (Figure 15–4b). Both hands should be brought together as the axe hits the wood. Separate the hands again on the stroke back up over your shoulder (Figure 15–4c). To cut a tree branch, make a sharp diagonal cut down first and follow with a second cut up. Repeat.

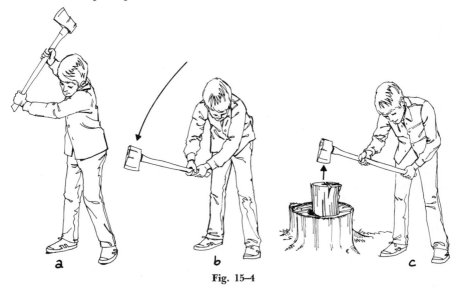

a   b   c

Fig. 15–4

Knives. Grasp a single- or double-blade knife in one hand with the thumb around it. Whittle away from you (Figure 15–5). Turn a stick and cut each new edge to point it. Cut a V notch. Make fuzz stick for fire tinder by starting about two inches from one end and cut down making long, thin strips.

Things to make from native materials with the axe, hatchet, and knife are:

Clothespins
Candlesticks
Belt buckles
Napkin rings
Book Covers
Sign posts and bulletin boards

Camp furniture
Wooden buttons
Letter openers
Green-stick cookers, broilers, pothooks, and other cooking aids

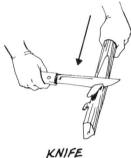

KNIFE
Fig. 15–5

SHELTERS

Outdoor living is best when one is comfortable. It is important to pick a good place to camp; there must be access to water, fuel, shade, and drainage in case of rain. These needs are all the more vital when dealing with handicapped people. Of course, outdoor living and sleeping, as well as other camping activities, must be geared to the physical, emotional, and mental condition of the people involved. As has been repeated many times, the leader must fully know the condition and needs of those he or she is teaching so that they can receive maximum benefit from the program.

A good bedroll is made of waterproof canvas, a poncho, a plastic tablecloth, and as many blankets as needed. Wool blankets are superior to cotton. The bedroll should be made so that the camper has as much cover beneath as above, for the ground gets cold during the night. The roll should be placed on a grassy spot free from rocks for sleeping. Pine needles, spruce, balsam, palmetto leaves, grass, ferns, and moss make an excellent mattress. A mosquito net supported by sticks and string will add to sleeping comfort. Beginners and handicapped persons should sleep in some kind of shelter before trying to sleep outdoors under the sky.

Outdoor shelters such as pup tents, poncho tents, lean-tos, cabins, tepees, tree houses, and tents all make good shelters (Figure 15–6). A canoe

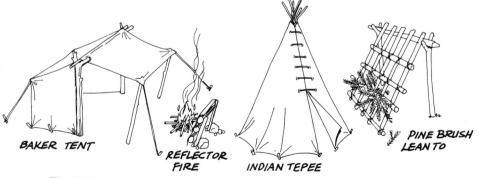

BAKER TENT   **REFLECTOR FIRE**   **INDIAN TEPEE**   **PINE BRUSH LEAN TO**

Fig. 15–6

turned on one side with the bottom facing outward can also be used. A brush den can be made and used as a last resort. Such a den can be quickly made by leaning a few poles against a log and covering them with boughs.

The most popular tent for permanent camps is the wall tent, named because of its upright canvas side walls. Guy ropes are used to tighten and loosen the tent; a clove hitch knot tied to a peg can be used if there are no tent adjustors.

A baker tent is recommended for winter use. With its front wide open to the warmth of a reflector fire it can be used by as many as four sleepers.

HIKING

A hike is a walk with a purpose. It is one of our few remaining cost-free recreational activities, and it is a good physical conditioner as well. There are many kinds of hikes, ranging from bird walks to mountain climbing. Many of the disabled can participate in this aspect of outdoor life with great pleasure and benefit.

Hikes should be carefully planned and should end at a choice spot. This serves as a group incentive. Singing and round-robin storytelling furnish fun along the way. Cookouts add to the joy of the hike's end. These should be simple meals such as toasted sandwiches, fried eggs and bacon, etc. All hikers must wear comfortable clothing. Laced oxfords and heavy wool socks are recommended. Distances can be gradually increased as the hikers gain stamina. Photography, sketching, or impromptu dramatics can be interwoven into hiking trips for variety.

TELLING DIRECTIONS

The North Star always indicates north, and as long as stars are shining one need not lose his way in the woods. The sun marks east and west by day. When the sky is overcast, however, the camper must use woods signs to find directions. These are:

Tree moss. There is usually more of it on the north side. Also, the moss grows highest there. Look at several trees before reaching your decision as to direction.

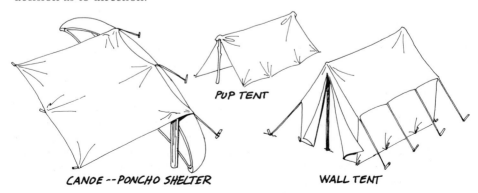

CANOE -- PONCHO SHELTER   PUP TENT   WALL TENT

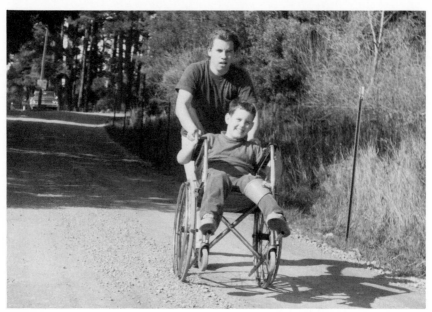

Hiking at camp can be done in many ways. Courtesy of the AAHPER.

Tree tops. The highest twigs of pines, spruces, and hemlocks usually lean a little east. Pick a tree in the open or the highest one in the area.

White paper. Your fingernail will do, if no paper is available. Stand in a clearing, hold a match upright on the paper and watch where the shadow falls. This will tell you your direction east from west, depending upon the time of day.

Watch. Hold the watch face up, place a match at the outer edge at the end of the hour hand. Turn the watch until the shadow of the match falls along the hour hand. In the a.m. south will be halfway, clockwise, between the hour hand and twelve o'clock. At noon the hour hand will point straight south. In the p.m. south will be half way, counterclockwise, between the hour hand and 12 o'clock.

Compass. Every camper going into the woods should carry one. Directions telling how to use it come in the box.

FISHING

This is an extremely popular American sport. It is a relatively inexpensive sport for beginners and it can be enjoyed in particular by many handicapped people because of its relative simplicity, its physically undemanding qualities, and its potential for relaxation.

Casting, both with a rod and reel, can be taught to beginners of mixed age in a gymnasium or any other large room. A skilled leader who knows the value of group organization can teach as many as fifty persons arranged in subgroups or squads. One group can practice stringing the line, another casting, a third tying flies, a fourth studying pictures and charts showing the habits of certain fish. Everyone should be doing something to learn about this fascinating and satisfying sport.

Skilled casters should assist the leader, be organized into casting

clubs, taken on fishing trips, shown how to improve their skills, or encouraged to compete in local, state, or national contests.

Targets best suited for beginners meeting inside can be made from
heavy white cardboard cut into solid circles. These should be supported
behind by wooden blocks or in some other way. Those learning outside
at a pool, lake, or stream will find suitable targets in white painted bicycle
or car tires, wood or plastic rims. If possible, each person should furnish
his own equipment. Each should also be instructed in how to buy and
care for his own gear.

Bait casting is done with live, artificial, or fresh bait. Worms, spoons,
or port rind are often used. The rod is made from wood, steel, glass, or
bamboo.

Hold the rod easily in one hand with the thumb on the spool where
it feels best as you apply pressure to control the speed of the lure. Do
the overhead cast on three counts as shown in Figure 15–7.

1. Hold the rod almost horizontally.
2. Bring it back to an imaginary twelve, then one o'clock.
3. Snap your wrist, bringing the rod back down slightly above your original
   horizontal position.

Practice to develop a smooth, relaxed, accurate cast. Use the rod tip for
aiming, and whip the line straight ahead each time. Avoid back casting

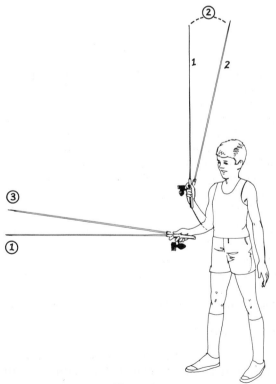

Fig. 15–7

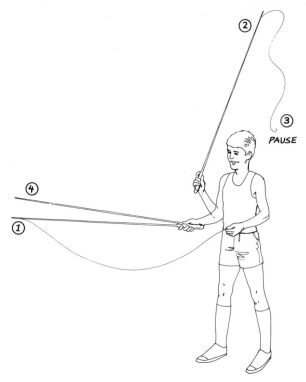

Fig. 15–8

too far on tensing up. Stand squarely, or with the opposite leg forward in a stride position (right leg forward for a left-handed person and vice versa for a right-handed one).

Fly casting is done with artificial or live bait. Artificial flies are multicolored and have colorful names such as the royal coachman, grizzly bear, etc. Live bait includes salmon eggs, worms, grasshoppers, and minnows. The rod is made from tubular steel, split bamboo, or glass.

Hold the rod easily in one hand with the thumb on top or at one side (whichever is more comfortable). Learn to cast on four counts as shown in Figure 15–8.

1. Hold the rod horizontally; take up the line slack with an outward pull of the opposite hand.
2. Snap the line back over your head to one o'clock.
3. Make a momentary pause until the lure completes its backward movement.
4. Snap the rod almost back down to its original horizontal position.

HORSEBACK RIDING

There is something magical about horseback riding, for the handicapped person as well as the normal. Polio victims, spastics, the blind,

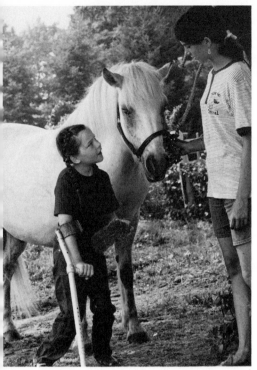 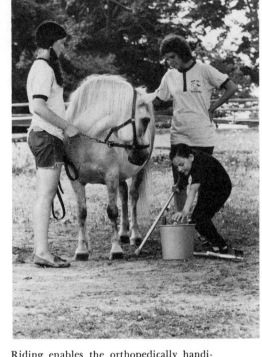

Horses can help the handicapped reduce their concentration on themselves and/or disillusionment with life. Courtesy of the National Foundation for Happy Horsemanship for the Handicapped, Inc.

Riding enables the orthopedically handicapped to learn the joy of free movement. Courtesy of the National Foundation for Happy Horsemanship for the Handicapped, Inc.

deaf, and emotionally disturbed especially find such experiences a thrilling adventure.[4]

Riding helps children gain confidence. It also helps them gain a feeling of independence. There seems to be a particular empathy between handicapped children and ponies—especially the autistic. Learning to ride has in some cases even produced speech in an otherwise speechless child. Riding teachers have noticed a general overall improvement in the learning attempts of disabled children.

Physically, many children, having discovered that the pony is providing the needed balance, learn to relax parts of their bodies controlled by tight muscles. Their general health improves from exercising in fresh air. Moreover, there is often an exchange between helpers and children, with the pony as a common ground.

Riding should be taught at camp on a one-to-one basis, using one helper for each child. Such assistants should have a training period given by the class instructor before they actually begin working with the handicapped. Horseback riding, as well as contact with other animals,

4 Miss Maudie Hunter-Warfel (Mon Ami Le Cheval, Box 462, Malvern, Pa., 19355) can be contacted for information about the National Foundation for Happy Horsemanship for the Handicapped, Inc. She is the national advisor of this organization and has taught numerous handicapped people to ride well.

is indeed one of the fruitful areas of providing atypical individuals with physical and recreational education.

All of the above campcraft skills can be taught in small or large groups. Contests between squads or teams can serve as a means of learning as well as of evaluating the degree and speed of skill mastery. Groups will enjoy the following contests:

> Water boiling
> Fire building—with or without matches
> Wood chopping
> Lashing camp tables, bridges, etc.
> Whittling
> Making functional crafts from native materials
> Pie, cookie, or cake baking contests
> Casting to targets placed at varied distances
> Biggest fish caught
> Fishing for the most fish
> Knotcraft displays
> Tent pitching and ditching for speed
> Trail blazing

NEEDED EQUIPMENT

Enjoyable camping is comfortable camping. Having the proper and necessary equipment with you adds to the luxury of outdoor living and sharpens its pleasure. Suggested equipment for a camp of four to six persons includes:

> *For Cooking*
> 1 pail for boiling water
> 1 kettle for sterilizing dishes
> 2 large cans with lids for drinking
> 4 kettles with lids
> 2 frying pans
> 1 dish pan
> 1 mixing bowl
> 2 large cooking spoons
> 1 pancake turner
> 1 butcher knife
> 2 peeling knives
> 1 salt shaker
> 1 pepper shaker
> 1 complete table service for each camper
>
> *Miscellaneous*
> 1 lantern
> 1 flashlight
> 1 jar of kitchen matches
> 1 first-aid kit

4 dish towels
2 dish rags
1 box of soap flakes or 2 bars of laundry soap
toilet paper
paper napkins
rope
rubber bands

Tools

1 large axe
2 small hatchets
1 short-handled shovel
1 buck saw

CLOTHING

Jeans, dungarees, or Levis are most suitable for camp. Other items to take along are:

Shorts
A wool or flannel shirt with long sleeves
A cotton shirt with long sleeves
Socks
Underclothing
Pajamas
Two pairs of comfortable hiking shoes (oxfords or laced heavy shoes preferred)
A rain coat and rain hat
A sweater
A wool or leather jacket
Bathing suit and cap

Optional personal items to take along include:

Books
Toilet articles (comb, brush, miror, etc.)
Pencil, paper, envelopes
Toothbrush and paste
Pocket knife
Linen (sheets, blankets, pillow)
A camera
A small musical instrument (harmonica, ukulele, etc.)
A deck of cards

LEADERSHIP

The key person in camp is the counselor. This person must be a combination of parent, friend, social worker, and teacher. Above all, the counselor must realize his or her important role in providing a model for young people.

Qualities, both professional and personal, necessary for camp counselors are:

1. A basic understanding of self, others, and the principles of group living
2. Resourcefulness, emotional stability, and creativity
3. Sense of humor, responsibility, and values
4. A belief in people and a desire to work with them
5. A zest for life, and the ability to capitalize and use constructively the enthusiasm and idealism of youth
6. Enjoyment of, and adaptability to outdoor life and group living
7. Basic camping skills

All counselors must be warm, mature people who truly love nature, camping, and the out-of-doors. Those working with the handicapped must have a thorough knowledge of teaching principles *and* of the disabilities and needs of their charges. Even junior counselors should have unusual ability and empathy for the handicapped. A ratio of three campers to one general counselor is recommended. All staff must have special skills needed for the handling of campers with certain types of disabilities. These abilities include lifting, dressing, feeding, toileting, putting on prosthetic and orthotic devices such as braces, splints, and artificial limbs, safe handling of wheelchairs, and an understanding of the special needs and limitations of the handicap they will deal with.

The total camp staff should include a director, unit or subgroup leaders, general and specialty leaders, junior counselors and/or counselors-in-training, health personnel, and maintenance men. The number of leaders will depend upon the size of the camp.

Camp directors are becoming increasingly aware of the importance of training their own staffs. Although many counselors have received general camp training elsewhere, each director should give specific training to his staff. The content of the training program depends greatly upon the disabilities that will be involved.

This complete training program should contain five elements: (1) the before-camp training, which takes place away from camp during three or more months prior to camp opening; (2) the pre-camp training at the camp before the campers arrive; (3) the in-service or continuous training, which goes on throughout the season; (4) the post-season evaluation period, and (5) the counselor-in-training program for older youth.

All training programs should be built around the broad areas of (1) the philosophy, aims, and objectives of the camp; (2) camping as a means of education and worthy use of leisure time; (3) health and safety rules and procedure; (4) individual and group guidance techniques; (5) methods of democratic leadership; (6) job analysis; and (7) campcraft skills.

It has been said that youth is a bank in which adults deposit their most precious treasures—their hard-won wisdom and their dreams of a better, happier, more secure world. All the accomplishments of tomorrow will be judged by the type of education young people receive today—and this certainly includes disabled youth. The summer camp, whether it is operated on a short- or long-term basis, or is publicly or privately owned, has taken its rightful place beside our other recognized educational institutions—the home, the school, and the church. It is important to realize that camping should help youth and adults live more abundantly, now and tomorrow. As leader-teachers, camping leaders deal with America's most precious possession—her children.

The Counselor as Educator

Counselor must realize the importance of the basic principles of learning, and fully apply those principles in the camp. Their chief function as leaders is to teach children *through* activities. To best utilize the camp environment, the counselor must know and enjoy campcraft skills. He should select with campers those activities that are fun, educationally challenging, and satisfying for each person and each group.

The daily, weekly, and seasonal programs should be evaluated periodically by campers, counselors, and the director. This may be done by group discussions, individual conferences, and observations. The best evidence of the effectiveness of the program will be gathered from observing the campers. If they are happy and have been challenged to become better functioning individuals and group members; if they exhibit changes in behavior, attitudes, and interests; and if they are aware of their importance as citizens in the camp community, the camp program has been effective and educational.

SUGGESTED READINGS

American Camping Association, *Resident Camp Standards; Day Camp Standards; Family Camp Standards.* Bradford Woods, Martinsville, Ind., 1975.

Boy Scouts of America, *Camping; Conservation in Camping; Firemanship; Forestry; Knots and How to Tie Them; Pioneering; Hiking; Orienteering; Boy Scout Field Book; Whittling; Woodcarving; Cooking; Weather.* New Brunswick, N.J.: 1973.

Easter Seal, *Guide to Special Camping Programs* (1970). 2023 West Odgen Avenue, Chicago, Illinois 60612.

Girl Scouts of America, *Girl Scout Handbook; Flip Charts of Campcraft Skills; Compass and Maps; Toolcraft; Knife and Axe; Let's Start Cooking; Working with the Handicapped, A Leader's Guide* (1973). 830 Third Avenue, New York, N.Y.

MITCHELL, GRACE, *Fundamentals of Day Camping.* New York: Association Press, 1961.

MITCHELL, VIOLA, IDA B. CRAWFORD, and JULIA ROBBERSON, *Camp Counseling,* 5th ed. Philadelphia: W. B. Saunders, 1975.

National Association for Retarded Children, *Day Camping for the Mentally Retarded* (1974). 420 Lexington Avenue, New York, N. Y. 10017.

SCHOENBOHN, WILCO, *Planning and Operating Facilities for Crippled Children.* Springfield,Ill.: Charles Thomas, 1974.

SHUTTLEWORTH, DOROTHY, *Exploring Nature with Your Child.* New York: Greystone Press, 1957.

U.S. Bureau of Recreation, *Outdoor Recreation for the Handicapped.* Washington, D.C.: Superintendent of Documents, *Technical Assistance Bulletin* (April 1967), 1973.

16

Professional Growth

Preliminary professional preparation and leadership experiences are basic to gaining effective results when working with all people, but especially so for those teaching the handicapped. Although professional preparation programs have greatly improved for these specialized leaders over the last decade, there remains a great lack of qualified leaders today. State education departments and colleges and universities are increasingly requiring internship experiences for graduation as well as for certification and further graduate study.

Tomorrow's leaders must be even more knowledgeable and skilled than are their colleagues of today. They must find ways to put into practice the results of the many current research projects as well as do meaningful research on their own. The population explosion, increased urbanization, a longer life span, increased leisure time, and world and individual tension all make the continued problem of dealing with the handicapped ever more important. The future for special education, corrective and/or adaptive physical education, and therapeutic recreation will only be as promising as the developing leaders.

Four ways for the leader to grow professionally are through self-evaluation, improved programs of supervision and internship, in-service improvement programs, and further education.

GROWTH THROUGH SELF-EVALUATION

It is not easy to judge oneself or the effectiveness of one's work realistically. Yet this is basic to self-improvement. No one is born a skilled leader; this status can only be attained by trial and error. Socrates' counsel of "Know thyself" is a lifelong quest, as is the obtaining of an education, for learning is a "must" as long as there is life. Experience is no real value unless one profits from it.

Most people wish at times that they had chosen another profession. There are moments, too, when all leaders get discouraged and feel they are not making progress. Those who are now in, or about to enter, a professional life of working with the handicapped might well give serious consideration to the following questions:

Why have you chosen this profession? To be of service, to make money, because nothing better turned up, for curiosity sake, because someone you admire is handicapped or works with the atypical? Are there other reasons?
What are your real professional plans and goals?
How long do you hope to remain in this profession?

The following self-appraisal check sheet should be filled out yearly by every leader interested in self-improvement and fulfillment. It should also be filled out by the supervisor and used for a follow-up personal conference geared toward professional growth.

Leader Self-Appraisal Check Sheet

Personal Qualities and Performance	*Consistently*	*Frequently*	*Need to work on this*
A. RELATIONSHIP WITH OTHERS			
1. Has good relationship with handicapped groups and the individuals in them.			
2. Has the respect and admiration of students and co-workers.			
3. Contributes a fair share to the success of group endeavor.			
4. Is respected and valued for professional contributions by superiors.			
B. APPEARANCE AND MANNER			
5. Is well-dressed and poised.			
6. Is emotionally mature.			
7. Is worthy of emulation by students and colleagues.			
8. Looks and acts the part of a leader.			
C. LEADERSHIP SKILLS			
9. Gives individual attention and help to each group member.			
10. Uses democratic leadership methods and develops leadership skills in each group.			

Personal Qualities and Performance	*Consistently*	*Frequently*	*Need to work on this*
11. Makes the most productive use of each class period.			_____
12. Teaches something new each class period.			_____
13. Has definite aims, goals, and objectives in mind.			_____
14. Makes the best use of every class period, facilities, and equipment.			_____
15. Provides a program which has variety, meaning, and carryover value.			_____
D. PROFESSIONAL QUALITIES			
16. Shows good professional judgment in decisions and actions.			_____
17. Works toward raising professional goals locally and nationally.			_____
18. Is continually growing professionally through study and research.			_____
19. Belongs and contributes to state, district, and local professional organizations.			_____
20. Deserves professional promotion and salary increases.			_____

PROGRAMS OF SUPERVISION AND INTERNSHIP

The internship experience should be geared to meet each student's needs and include contacts with as many program activities as possible, working with varying age groups from different socioeconomic backgrounds in a variety of settings, including hospitals, clinics, schools, and treatment centers.

To be most effective, all internship experiences should be carefully chosen and well-supervised. It is imperative that the supervisor be a master teacher-leader and that this internship experience cover a wide range of experiences. Because this laboratory-type experience is so valuable, it should come early in the sequence of professional preparation and be given for a long time period. The young intern should be encouraged to experiment and to observe learned theories under the supervision of an experienced teacher who can help the student profit from trial and error learning attempts.

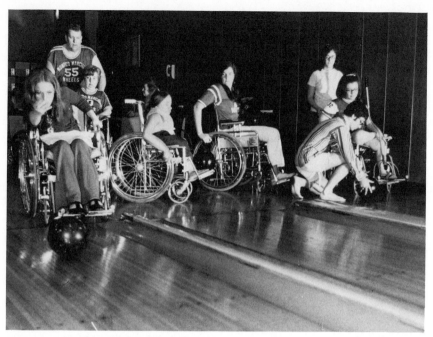

The professional preparation program for the adapted physical educator should include practical experiences as well as educational theory. Courtesy of the AAHPER.

The supervisor should have many private counseling sessions with each interning student. All should be carefully guided; they must learn to accept failure as a means of developing leadership skills. As a result of counseling sessions each student should become aware that his other primary role is to learn the profession, as well as how to work skillfully with others—and not merely to satisfy the supervisor in hope of gaining a glowing reference for a future position or receiving a good grade.

IN-SERVICE IMPROVEMENT PROGRAMS

In-service training is a self-improvement program. Staff meetings democratically led can be a rich source of growing in understanding and appreciation as well as gaining knowledge of current happenings. Because no person can learn for another, each staff member should be encouraged to try out individually the many new materials and ideas discussed in staff meetings. Professional growth is the continuous and personal responsibility of each physical activities leader. As a result of staff meetings, professionals working with the handicapped should improve in their performance as well as in relation to co-workers and the general public.

Faculty meetings should be held monthly (or more frequently as the need arises) in order to study instructional and administrative issues as well as share new information with professional colleagues. By participating fully in such meetings, each leader can improve working conditions, raise professional standards, and help mold the best kind of an educational program for the benefit of those taking part in it.

Suggested questions for staff members to ask themselves in regard to in-service staff meetings are:

1. Do you readily accept helpful suggested ways for upgrading your own professional status and that of your group?
2. Do you try out most of the new ideas, techniques, and materials presented in staff meetings?
3. Are your relations with your co-workers professional, cooperative, and friendly?
4. Do you profit from sharing experiences with older, more experienced leaders?
5. Do you make meaningful contribution toward the success of each staff meeting?

Staff meetings should generate professional enthusiasm and cooperation among all members. Discussion of current professional problems, the development of new materials and teaching methods, and reports of professional meetings should be the major agenda of such meetings. If the staff is to work as a team, it must share in making decisions that concern all the leaders as well as those they serve. Likewise, the staff should feel responsible for carrying out decisions made by the majority.

FURTHER EDUCATION

The saying, "the more you know, the more you realize how little you know," is true. Education never stops. Although continued education is costly, it yields many rich returns. It is a must for those who wish to teach at advanced levels or become leaders in their fields.

Those who wish to go on beyond the Master's level can receive either the Doctor of Philosophy degree (the Ph.D.) or the Doctor of Education degree (the Ed.D.). Both degrees are similar (although the latter is a newer degree) in admission standards, matriculation procedures, and residence and time requirements. The Ph.D. is aimed largely at one specific area of knowledge and is geared largely for those primarily interested in research. The Ed.D. specializes in some area of education and is largely for those who wish to pursue teaching or careers in the various facets of education.

Many graduate teaching fellowships and assistantships, scholarships and loans are available for those interested in advanced study.

Graduate work greatly enhances the chances for professional advancement as well as increasing respect for one's chosen profession. Supervisory and administrative positions require even broader professional experience and graduate degrees.

The future is brighter for the handicapped when, leaders in the field of therapeutic rehabilitation are interested in professional growth and in fulfilling the needs of others. There is no doubt that this can be an exciting, challenging, and worthwhile lifetime occupation for men and women who have the capacity to serve others.

SUGGESTED READINGS

American Association for Health, Physical Education and Recreation, *Profes-sional Preparation in Health Education, Physical Education, and Recreation Education* (1962); *Directory of Professional Preparation Institutions* (1966); *Graduate Educational in Health Education, Physical Education, Recreation, Safety, and Dance* (1967). Washington, D.C.: AAHPER.

American Recreation Society, *Recreation in Treatment Centers*, Vol. 3. Washington, D.C.: American Recreation Society, 1964.

Northwest Regional Special Education Instructional Materials Center, *Catalog of Instructional Materials and Resource Materials for Teaching and Learning with Handicapped Children and Youth.* Eugene, Oregon: Clinical Services, University of Oregon, 1975.

Appendices

APPENDIX A

Professional Organizations

American Alliance for Health, Physical Education and Recreation
    (a department of the National Education Association)
    1201 16th Street, N.W., Washington, D.C. 20036

American Medical Association
    535 North Dearborn Street, Chicago, Illinois 60610

American Occupational Therapy Association, Inc.
    3310 East 42nd Street, New York, N.Y. 10017

American Physical Therapy Association
    1790 Broadway, New York, New York 10019

American Psychiatric Association
    1700 18th Street, N.W., Washington, D.C. 20036

American Psychological Association
    1333 16th Street, N.W., Washington, D.C. 20036

American Speech Correction Association
    Speech and Hearing Clinic
    (headquarters changes annually to location of elected secretary-treasurer)

International Council for Exceptional Children
    1201 16th Street, N.W., Washington, D.C. 20036

National Foundation
    1790 Broadway, New York, N.Y. 10019

National Rehabilitation Association
    1025 Vermont Avenue, Washington, D.C. 20005

APPENDIX B

Societies and Associations

American Federation of the Physically Handicapped, Inc.
1376 National Press Building, Washington, D.C. 20004

American Hearing Society
817 14th Street, N.W., Washington, D.C. 20005

American Heart Association, Inc.
1790 Broadway, New York, N.Y. 10019

American Legion National Rehabilitation Committee
1608 K Street, N.W., Washington, D.C. 20006

Association for the Aid of Crippled Children
345 East 46th Street, New York, N.Y. 10017

Children's Bureau, Department of Health, Education and Welfare
Washington, D.C. 20014

Comeback, Inc.
16 West 46th Street, New York, N.Y. 10036

Dallas Association for Retarded Children
3121 N. Harwood St., Dallas, Texas 75201

Dallas Services for Blind Children, Inc.
3802 Cole Ave., Dallas, Texas 75204

Goodwill Industries of America, Inc.
744 N. 4th Street, Milwaukee, Wisconsin 53201

Institute for the Crippled and Disabled
400 1st Avenue, New York, N.Y. 10010

Muscular Dystrophy Association of America, Inc.
1790 Broadway, New York, N.Y. 10019

National Association for Mental Health
10 Columbus Circle, New York, N.Y. 10019

National Council on Rehabilitation
1790 Broadway, New York, N.Y. 10019

National Epilepsy League
208 North Wells Street, Chicago, Illinois 60606

National Organization for Mentally Ill Children
171 Madison Avenue, New York, N.Y. 10010

National Society for Crippled Children and Adults, Inc.
11 South LaSalle Street, Chicago, Illinois 60603

National Society for the Prevention of Blindness, Inc.
1790 Broadway, New York, N.Y. 10019

National Tuberculosis Association
    1790 Broadway, New York, N.Y. 10019

Scottish Rite Hospital for Crippled Children
    2201 Welborn St., Dallas, Texas 75219

United Cerebral Palsy Association
    50 West 57th Street, New York, N.Y. 10019

United States Office of Education, Department of Health, Education and Welfare
    Washington, D.C. 20202

Vocational Rehabilitation Administration, Department of Health, Education and
    Welfare, Washington, D.C. 20202

Volta Bureau
    1537 35th Street, N.W., Washington, D.C. 20007

APPENDIX C

Periodicals

American Heart Journal
American Journal of Hygiene
American Journal of Occupational Therapy
American Journal of Physiology
American Journal of Public Health
Archives of Pediatrics
Archives of Physical Medicine and Rehabilitation
Child Development
Journal of the American Dietetic Association
Journal of the Association for Physical and Mental Rehabilitation
Journal of Bone and Joint Surgery
Journal of Exceptional Children
Journal of Health, Physical Education and Recreation
Mental Hygiene
Physical Educator
Physical Therapy Review
Physiotherapy
Recreation
Recreation in Treatment Centers
Rehabilitation Record
Research Quarterly
Today's Health

Adapted Exercise Gymnasium and Recreation Equipment List
(Large Facility)

REMEDIAL EXERCISE EQUIPMENT

Stationary Equipment

Single-section stall bars
Stall bar chinning bar
Triplex wall pulley weights
Shoulder wheel
Pronator-supinator machine
Wall horizontal bar
Adjustable height striking bag
Shoulder ladder

Stall bar bench
Floor and chest pulley weights
Latissimus Dorsi exerciser
Wrist roll machine
Multi-chinning bar
Horizontal ladder
Peg climb board
Stationary arm-leg-hip whirlpool

Movable Equipment

Elgin exercise unit
Footstool
Heavy duty N-K unit
Rowing machine
Training bag
Ankle and leg exerciser

Exercise table
Abdominal incline board
Treadmill with handrails
Bicycle exerciser
Densifoam gym mat

Posture Training Area

Posture training mirror, stationary
Movable posture training mirror
Posture grid screen and evaluation kit

Adjustable sitting posture training stool
Foot inversion tread
Arthrodial protractor

Resistance Training Equipment

Dumbbell wagon with dumbbells
Muscle-matic kit
Barbell set and weights
Medicine ball
Quadriceps boot with bar and collars
Wrist cuff
Ankle cuff
Shoulder strap
Tension hand grips

Weight caddy with disc-type weights
Sandbag set
Press bench
Medicine ball rack
Foot stirrup
Thigh cuff
Head strap
Back weight pan
Grip exerciser

Group Exercise Equipment

Cage ball   Wands with wand rack
Indian clubs   Indian club hangers
Exer-gym   Spring pull exerciser
Rubber exerciser   Jumprope
Balance board

Testing, Measurement, and Anthropometric Devices

Body-weight scale   Dry spirometer
Lange skinfold caliper   Gulick anthropometric tape
Flexometer   Shoulder breadth caliper
Chest-depth caliper   Transparent goniometer
Hand dynamometer   Push-pull attachment for dynamometer
Back, leg, and chest dynamometer   Stopwatch
Timer   Electric rhythm metronome

Gymnastic Equipment

Low balance beam   Balance beam
Low parallel bar   Parallel bar
Trampoline   Mini-tramp
Side horse   Climbing rope
Still rings

Recreation Area

Gym scooter set   Shuffleboard set, indoor
Table tennis table   Scoopball kit
Tetherball set   Combination volleyball/badminton set
Lightweight bowling set   Rubber horseshoe set
Rubber quoit set   Professional hockey set
Beanbag game   Suction dart game
Croquet set   Paddle-racket set
Fun balls   Safe-T play bats
Nok hockey set   Cage balls

APPENDIX E

Adapted Exercise Room

(Small Facility)

REMEDIAL EXERCISE EQUIPMENT

Stationary Equipment

Single-section stall bars
Stall bar chinning bar
Triplex wall pulley weights
Shoulder wheel
Pronator-supinator machine
Wall horizontal bar
Horizontal ladder
Shoulder ladder

Stall bar bench
Floor and chest pulley weights
Latissimus Dorsi exerciser
Wrist roll machine
Multi-chinning bar
Horizontal bar
Peg climb board
Adjustable height striking bag

Movable Equipment

Elgin exercise unit
Footstool
Heavy-duty N-K unit
Rowing machine
Densifoam mat with mat hooks

Exercise table
Abdominal incline boards
Treadmill with handrails
Bicycle exerciser
Ankle and leg exerciser

Posture Training Area

Posture training mirror, stationary
Foot inversion tread
Arthrodial protractor

Adjustable sitting posture training stool
Posture grid screen and evaluation kit

Resistance Training Equipment

Dumbbell set
Weight caddy with disc-type weights
Sandbag set
Press bench
Quadriceps boot with bar and collars
Wrist cuff
Ankle cuff
Shoulder strap
Tension hand grips

Dumbbell rack
Muscle-matic kit
Barbell set and weights
Medicine ball with ball rack
Foot stirrup
Thigh cuff
Head strap
Back weight pan
Grip exerciser

Group Exercise Equipment

Cage ball   Wands with rack
Indian clubs   Indian club hangers
Exer-gym   Spring pull exerciser
Rubber exerciser   Jumprope
Balance board

Testing, Measurement, and Anthropometric Devices

Body-weight scale   Dry spirometer
Lange skinfold caliper   Gulick anthropometric tape
Flexometer   Shoulder breadth caliper
Chest-depth caliper   Transparent goniometer
Hand dynamometer   Push-pull attachment for dynamometer
Back, leg, and chest dynamometer   Stopwatch
Exercise timer   Electric rhythm metronome

Recreation Area

Lightweight bowling set   Horseshoe set
Rubber quoit set   Beanbag game
Suction dart game   Croquet set
Nok hockey set

Gymnastic Equipment

Low balance beam   Side horse
Still rings   Climbing ropes

APPENDIX F

Developmental Elementary Gymnasium

Stationary Equipment

Single-section stall bars
Stall bar chinning bar
Walking ramp
Multi-chinning bar
Posture training mirror, stationary
Still rings
Bicycle exerciser

Stall bar bench
Horizontal bar
Staircase, corner type
Peg climb board
Climbing rope
Shoulder wheel

Movable Equipment

Bicycle exerciser
Adjustable height striking bag
Low parallel bars
Trampoline

Training bag
Low balance beam
Side horse
Densifoam mat

Resistance Training Equipment

Dumbbell set
Muscle-matic kit
Medicine ball

Child-size quadriceps boot
Sandbag set
Medicine ball rack

Group Exercise Equipment

Scooter board
Cage ball
Indian club
Rubber exerciser
Balance board

Maxie club
Wands with rack
Indian club hangers
Jumprope

Testing, Measurement, and Anthropometric Devices

Body-weight scale
Lange skinfold caliper
Flexometer
Chest-depth caliper
Hand dynamometer
Timer

Dry spirometer
Gulick anthropometric tape
Shoulder breadth caliper
Transparent goniometer
Stopwatch
Electric rhythm metronome

Recreation Area

Gym scooter set
Table tennis table
Tetherball set
Rubber horseshoe set
Professional hockey set
Suction dart boards
Croquet set
Fun balls
Safe-T play bats

Shuffle board set, indoor
Scoop ball kit
Volleyball/badminton set
Rubber quoit set
Beanbag game
Nok hockey set
Paddle-racket set
Lightweight bowling set
Cage ball

APPENDIX G

Sources of Equipment and Supplies

Alberta's Ceramic Supply
5434 N. Peters Street
New Orleans, La. 70117

American Art Clay Co·
4717 W. 16th Street
Indianapolis, Ind. 46224

American Athletic Equipment Co.
Box 111
Jefferson, Ia. 50129

American Handicraft Co.
Advertising Department
1991 Foch Street
Fort Worth, Tex. 76102

American Reedcraft Corp.
417 LaFayette Street
Hawthorne, N.J. 07507

American Seating Co.
300 North Central Expressway
Dallas, Tex. 75080

The American Thread Co.
260 West Broadway
New York, N.Y. 10013

Archer Plastics, Inc.
1125 Close Ave.
Bronx, N.Y. 10472

The Arrow Rubber and Plastics
Box 104
West Englewood, N.J. 07666

Athletic Trainers Supply Co.
427 Broadway
New York, N.Y. 10013

Banner Plastics Corp.
80 Beckwith Ave.
Paterson, N.J. 07503

Barr Rubber Products Co.
Sandusky, O. 44870

Better Gift Service, Inc.
4505 Liberty Ave.
Pittsburgh, Pa. 15224

Stanley Bowmar Co., Inc.
12 Cleveland Street
Valhalla, N.Y. 10595

Milton Bradley Co.
Springfield, Mass. 01102

Broadhead Barret Co.
4560 East 71st Street
Cleveland, O. 44105

California Ceramics, Inc.
12422 East Carson Street
Artesia, Cal. 90701

Childcraft Equipment Co., Inc.
155 E. 23rd Street
New York, N.Y. 10110

Childhood Interest, Inc.
Factory—Roselle, N.J. 07203
Showroom—200 5th Ave.
New York, N.Y. 10010

Childplay of New York, Inc.
203 West 14th Street
New York, N.Y. 10011

Children's Music Center, Inc.
5373 West Pico Blvd.
Los Angeles, Cal. 90019

Community Playthings
Rifton, N.Y. 12471

Cooperative Recreation Service, Inc.
Radnor Road
Delaware, O. 43015

H. Davis Toy Corp.
794 Union Street
Brooklyn, N.Y. 11215

Diamond Yarn Corp.
10 West 29th Street
New York, N.Y. 10001

Game-Time, Inc.
Littlefield, Mich. 49252

Geant Manufacturing Co.
Council Bluffs, Ia. 51501

General Playground Equipment Co.
1139 South Courtland Avenue
Kokomo, Ind. 46901

The Gong Bell Mfg. Co.
200 5th Ave.
New York, N.Y. 10010

325

J. L. Hammett Co.
Cambridge, Mass. 02139

Frederick Herrschner
72 E. Randolph Street
Chicago, Ill. 60601

Holland Mold, Inc.
1040 Pennsylvania Ave.
Trenton, N.J. 08608

House of Ceramics, Inc.
2481 Matthews
Memphis, Tenn. 38108

The House of Wood and Crafts
3408 12 North Holton Street
Milwaukee, Wisc. 53212

Ideal Toy Corp.
200 5th Ave.
New York, N.Y. 10010

Irwin Corp.
85 Factory St.
Nashua, N.H. 03060

Alan Jay
3547 Webster Ave.
New York, N.Y. 10067

Jolly Toys, Inc.
459 West 15th St.
New York, N.Y. 10011

Kiln Paragon Industries
P.O. Box 10133
Dallas, Tex. 75207

Knickerbocker Toy Co.
1107 Broadway
New York, N.Y. 10010

Merribee Art Embroidery Co.
1515 University Dr.
Fort Worth, Tex. 76102

National Handicraft Co., Inc.
199 Williams St.
New York, N.Y. 10038

Norman Ceramics Co., Inc.
Mamaroneck, N.Y. 10543

Playground Corp. of America
29-16 40th Rd.
Long Island City, N.Y. 11101

Playground Equipment
The Mexico Forge, Inc.
Mexico, Pa. 17056

Playtime Products, Inc.
Warsaw, Ind. 46580

Port-a-Pit Co.
P.O. Box C
Temple City, Cal. 91780

Practical Drawing Co.
P.O. Box 5388
Dallas, Tex. 75222

J. A. Preston Co.
71 5th Ave.
New York, N.Y. 10003

Program Aids, Inc.
161 McQuesten Parkway
Mt. Vernon, N.Y. 10550

San Rubber Co.
Barberton, O. 44203

School Playthings, Inc.
109 West Hubbard St.
Chicago, Ill. 60610

Selected Equipment for School
    Activities
Beckley-Cardy School Buyers
1900 North Narragansett
Chicago, Ill. 60629

Stewart Clay Co., Inc.
333 Mulberry St.
New York, N.Y. 10013

Tandy Leather Co.
609 Laura Street
Jacksonville, Fla. 32702

Terrace Ceramic Supply
403 Sterlington Rd.
Monroe, La. 71201

Thrift Mailmart
Wantagh, N.Y. 11793

W. J. Voit Corp.
29 Essex Street
Maywood, N.J. 07607

Walco Toy Co., Inc.
38 W. 37th St.
New York, N.Y. 10108

Lee Wards
Liberty and Page Ave.
Elgin, Ill. 60120

Wolverine Sports Supply
3666 South State St.
Ann Arbor, Mich. 48108

APPENDIX H

Recommended Films and Filmstrips
for Class and Community Use

Cast No Shadow (16mm, color and sound). A film showing physically crippled and mentally retarded children engaged in a variety of recreational activities at the Recreation Center for the Handicapped in San Francisco. Professional Arts, Inc., Box 8484, Universal City, California 91608

New Concepts in Children's Play Areas (80 frames of filmstrip, sound and color, 20 minutes). The newest creative types of playground equipment are shown. These have been designed to meet children's developmental levels and needs. Associated Film Services, 3419 West Magnolia, Burbank, California 91505

Physical Education for Blind Children (16mm, color and sound, 28 minutes). Shows blind children playing many games and sports, including track and field events. Dr. Charles Buell, 4244 Health Rd., Long Beach, California 90808

Recreational Activities for Mentally Retarded Children (16mm, color and sound, 28 minutes). Film shows a wide variety of activities for the retarded, and includes outings and parties as well as crafts, music, and games. National Association for Retarded Children, 420 Lexington Avenue, New York, N.Y. 10017

Recreation for the Handicapped (16mm, color and sound, 23 minutes). Shows many recreational activities for all age groups with varying types of disabilities. Recreation Center for the Handicapped, Great Highway at Sloat Blvd., San Francisco, California 94132

The Therapeutic Community (16mm, sound and color, 28 minutes). Filmed in a geriatric hospital setting, this movie gives viewers insight into the many problems of the aged and scope of therapeutic teams available to assist them. University of Michigan Television Center and Division of Gerontology, Ann Arbor, Michigan

Therapy through play (16mm, sound and color, 17 minutes). This film shows how many sports and games can be adapted to fit the needs of physically disabled children. Human Resources Center, Albertson, N.Y. 11507

The following filmstrips on sports are available both for rental and purchase from the Athletic Institute, 805 Merchandise Mart, Chicago, Illinois 60654:

Apparatus Activities for Boys and Men
Archery
Badminton
Campcraft Shelters
Campcraft Series
Fishing
Gymnastics for Girls and Women
Lifesaving

327

THE CRIPPLED CHILD'S
"Bill of Rights"

THE International Society for Crippled Children, in Tenth Annual Convention assembled, at Cleveland, Ohio, declared the following to be the "Crippled Child's 'Bill of Rights,' " in which and through which the Society, for the first time states, from the standpoint of the child, its program for the prevention of crippling conditions, the finding of the crippled child, its care, treatment and education, and finally, its placement in the life of the World.

I   Every child has the right to be well born; that is to say, the right to a sound body, complete in its members, physically whole. In the securing of this right we pledge ourselves to use our influence that proper pre-natal, intra-natal and post-natal care be provided to the end that congenital deformity, insofar as it is humanly and scientifically possible, be prevented.

II   Every child has the right to develop under clean, wholesome, healthful conditions. In declaring this right, this Society undertakes to use its influence to the end that children everywhere, through proper legislation, both local and general, and through proper supervision and protection, may grow to manhood and womanhood free from crippling conditions caused by insufficient nourishment, improper food, or unsanitary environment, and free so far as possible, from danger of accident, wounding or maiming.

III   Notwithstanding the rights of children to be well born and to be protected throughout childhood, it is recognized that in spite of all human precautions there will be, unfortunately, some crippled children. These we declare to have the right to the earliest possible examination, diagnosis and treatment, recognizing, as we do, the fact that many thousand cases of permanent crippling may be eliminated by early and effective care.

IV   Every crippled child has a right, not only to the earliest possible treatment, but to the most effective continuing care, treatment and nursing, including the use of such appliances as are best calculated to assist in remedying or ameliorating its condition.

V   Every crippled child has the right to an education. Without this, all other provisions, unless for the relief of actual suffering, are vain.

VI   Every crippled child has the right not only to care, treatment and education, but to such treatment as will fit him or her for self-support, either wholly or partially, as the conditions may dictate. Without such practical application education is likewise purposeless.

VII   Every crippled child has the right to vocational placement, for unless the child,—boy or girl—after having been given physical care and treatment, and after being educated and trained, is actually placed in a proper position in the life of the World, all that has gone before is of no avail.

VIII   Every crippled child has the right to considerate treatment, not only from those responsible for its being and for its care, treatment, education and placement, but from those with whom it is thrown into daily contact, and every possible influence should be exerted by this and affiliated organizations to secure this right, in order that, so far as possible, the crippled child may be spared the stinging jibe or the bitter taunt, or, worse still, the demoralizing pity of its associates.

IX   Every crippled child has the right to spiritual, as well as bodily development, and, without regard to particular religious or denominational belief, is entitled to have nourishment for soul-growth.

X   In brief, not only for its own sake, but for the benefit of Society as a whole, every crippled child has the right to the best body which modern science can help it to secure; the best mind which modern education can provide; the best training which modern vocational guidance can give; the best position in life which his physical condition, perfected as best as it may be, will permit, and the best opportunity for spiritual development which its environment affords.

Index

Index

Handicapped, 3–4, 7–10
  children, 25–29
  recreational programs for, 10–15
Handicaps:
  auditory, 59–62
  cerebral palsy, 44–49
  mental illness, 88–97
  mental retardation, 37–42
  orthopedic, 64–85
  physical, 7–10
  in school children, 8
  social, 7–10
  visual, 51–59
Hard of hearing, 59 (*see also* Deaf)
Haun, Paul, 94
Head tilt, forward, 78
Health, evaluation of, 143–44
Hearing handicaps (*see* Auditory handicaps)
Hearing tests, 144
Heart disease, 124–25
Hernia, 126
Hiking, 297
Hockey, 161
Holiday celebrations, 11
Holmgren Wool Test for Color-Blindness, 144
Horseback riding, 300–302
Hot Ball, 232–33
Hot Time in the Old Town (dance), 269–70
Hyperopia, 51

I

Indian Club Guard Ball, 229
Insanity, defined, 90
Insurance, 161
Internship, programs, 309–11
Iowa Brace Test, 146
IQ and retardation, 39, 40

J

Journal of Health, Physical Education and Recreation, 179
Jump the Shot (game), 230

K

Kalvelis (dance), 276
Keep Away (game), 224
Keep it Up (game), 214–15
Kelly Foot Pain Test, 144
Kennedy Foundation, 38, 41
Keyhole Basketball, 224
Kick ball, rules for, 204
Kick for Distance, rules for, 205
Kick It and Run (game), 229
Kickover Ball, 205
Knives, use of, 295
Knowledge, evaluation of, 146–49
Kraus-Weber Floor-Touch Test, 146
Kraus-Weber Refined Posture Test, 144
Kyphosis, 77

L

Latcham Motor Achievement Test, 146
Leader(s), 11–15, 135, 182, 183
  camp, 303–5
  role of, 164–69
  training of, 92–93, 307–11
Leader's Club, 183
Learning, 167–74
Legislation, federal, 6–7
Lesson plans, 195–96
Liabilities, 161–62
Life span, and obesity, 98
Lifetime Sports Education Project, 234n
Line Bowling, 212
Line Dodgeball, 233
Line Soccer, 206
Locker rooms, 183–84
Locomotor activities, 253–55
Long Base (game), 210
Lordosis, 77–78, 80–81
LSD, 66

M

Males, 29
Malnutrition, 29
Manic-depressive psychosis, 90

INVENTORY 1983